PRAISE FOR
THE SELF-COMPASSION DIET

"If you're tired of losing weight and then regaining more, forget about starting that same-old diet tomorrow. Read this book today. *The Self-Compassion Diet* delivers what you truly crave—a simple, flexible, proven plan for transforming the way you live, breathe, and eat. Synthesizing current psychological theory, cutting-edge research, tried-and-true mindful-eating practices, and winning hypnotic suggestions, Jean Fain shows you how to find your best way to a healthy, sustainable weight."

STEVEN GURGEVICH, PhD, author of The Self-Hypnosis Diet

"Self-compassion is the only approach that works, and with Jean Fain's guidance, you will not only wake up out of addictive eating patterns, you will have a pathway to deep happiness and transformation. Filled with the basic elements of healing—mindfulness, heartfulness, psychological strategies, and relational support—this book is a real gem!"

TARA BRACH, PhD, author of Radical Acceptance

"Jean Fain's *The Self-Compassion Diet* offers a welcome and fresh approach to weight loss for the battle-weary dieter. You won't find any forbidden food lists or calorie-counting strategies in this book. What you will find is the missing ingredient in most weight-loss approaches: self-compassion, which has the power to transform every eating experience into something bright and positive in your life. Fain's engaging writing style, complete with mini-assessments, helpful practices, and case-studies, will help you say goodbye to dieting, once-and-for-all, and feel good in the process."

EVELYN TRIBOLE, MS, RD, author of Intuitive Eating

"This delightful handbook moves the diet conversation to a new level. The author, diet expert Jean Fain, gently unravels the mystery behind successful change—self-kindness—and weaves it into a wise, carefully organized, multifaceted, step-by-step approach to healthy eating. Allow the subtle message into your heart and see how your food habits change from the ground up."

CHRISTOPHER K. GERMER, PhD, author of
The Mindful Path to Self-Compassion

"*The Self-Compassion Diet* by Jean Fain blends Eastern meditative techniques and Western psychology for a gentle, comprehensive approach to weight loss. These techniques will help people of any weight to be calmer and happier with their lives."

DEIRDRE BARRETT, author *Supernormal Stimuli*

"This book translates an established research finding—that self-compassion is a more effective motivator than self-criticism—into a practical, easy-to-follow guide for losing weight. This book will not only transform your waistline, it will change your life."

KRISTIN NEFF, PhD, author of *Self-Compassion*

THE
SELF-
COMPASSION
DIET

THE SELF-COMPASSION DIET

A Step-by-Step Program
to Lose Weight with
Loving-Kindness

JEAN FAIN, LICSW, MSW

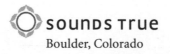

SOUNDS TRUE
Boulder, Colorado

Sounds True, Inc.
Boulder, CO 80306

Cover and book design by Karen Polaski

Satter, E. "What is normal eating?" Copyright © 2009 by Ellyn Satter. Published
at www.EllynSatter.com. For more about eating competence (and for research
backing up this advice), see Ellyn Satter's *Secrets of Feeding a Healthy Family: How
to Eat, How to Raise Good Eaters, How to Cook*, Kelcy Press, 2008. Also see www.
EllynSatter.com/shopping to purchase books and to review other resources.

The link to self-compassion scale, "How Self-Compassionate Are You?" (self-
compassion.org/how_self-compassionate_are_you.html) reprinted with
permission by Kristin Neff.

Printed in Canada

Library of Congress Cataloging-in-Publication Data

Fain, Jean.
The self-compassion diet : a step-by-step program to lose weight with loving-
kindness / Jean Fain.
    p. cm.
Includes bibliographical references.
ISBN 978-1-60407-075-0 (alk. paper)
1. Weight loss. 2. Compassion. 3. Psychotherapy. I. Title.
RM222.2.F28 2011
613.2'5—dc22
              2010026049

E-book ISBN 978-1-60407-326-3

10 9 8 7 6 5 4 3 2

Disclaimers
On identity: Clients agreed to share their stories if their identities were disguised.
On gender: Because diet-book readers are predominantly female, this book uses
many more female metaphors and pronouns than male. I welcome readers of
all genders, but too much unisex language hurts my writer's ears. If you're in the
male minority, please accept my apologies and keep reading. This weight-loss plan
delivers measurable results from day one—to men and women. If the metaphors
and pronouns don't fit, don't wear them. Feel free to mentally substitute words that
suit you better.
On health: If you suffer from a serious medical or psychological problem, the first
act of loving-kindness you'll need to practice is checking with your primary health
giver. If you've got a trauma history or a life-threatening eating disorder, don't try
these practices alone. Enlist the help of a trusted therapist. If you've got medical
concerns, including issues related to gastric bypass surgery, consult your doctor
before starting this or any eating program.

*In memory of my mother and
in appreciation of my husband.*

*Their boundless love and support
have made this book possible.*

CONTENTS

Preface: The Impatient Dieter xiii
Introduction: Planning Your Journey 1

PART I   Self-Compassion:
          The Power of Loving-Kindness
     1   The Kinder, Gentler Therapist. 11
     2   Loving-Kindness Suggestions for Cultivating Compassion . . 29

PART II   Hypnosis:
          The Power of Positive Suggestion
     3   The Enchanting Hypnotherapist. 53
     4   Winning Weight-Loss Suggestions for Staying Slim 73

PART III Mindfulness:
          The Power of Conscious Awareness
     5   The Curious Meditator. 103
     6   Mindful-Eating Suggestions for Savoring Each Bite . . . 129

PART IV   Social Support:
          The Power of Compassionate Community
     7   The Successful Weight-Loss Buddy. 159
     8   Community-Building Suggestions for Seeking Support. .187

PART V   Continuing Education:
          The Power of Personal Persistence
     9   Ultimate Suggestions for Filling Your Toolbox 215

          Afterword: The Compassionate Guide 225
          Acknowledgments. 229
          Notes 233
          Further Reading and Resources. 245
          About the Author 257

LIST OF PRACTICES AND OTHER USEFUL TOOLS

I Loving-Kindness Suggestions
   Metta: Loving-Kindness Meditation 35
   Compassionate Advisor: A Guided Visualization 38
   Compassionate Note to Self: A Writing Exercise 41
   Compassionate Glasses: A Guided Visualization 43
   Head-to-Toe Appreciation: A Guided Visualization 46
   Tonglen: Give-and-Take Meditation 48

II Winning Weight-Loss Suggestions
   Outstanding Suggestions 92
   Encouraging Words 93
   Baby-Step Appreciation 94
   Picture of Health. 95
   Mindless Memories 97
   Imaginary Triggers 99

III Mindful-Eating Suggestions
   Breathe—The Longer Practice 136
   Float—The Shorter Practice 138
   Mindless-Eating Meditation 141
   Hunger-Awareness Meditation 143
   Taste-Satisfaction Meditation 145
   Full-Body Fullness Scan 147
   All-Purpose Eating Meditation, Parts I and II . . 150 and 153

IV Community-Building Suggestions
   Present Company Included: A Writing Exercise 195
   A Blast From the Past: A Writing Exercise 198
   In Good Company: A Guided Visualization 200
   Worlds Apart: A Guided Visualization. 204

Future Support Now: A Writing Exercise 206
Good to Go: A Field Trip 209

V Ultimate Suggestions 215

VI Power Tools
Attainable Goal List 79
Food Logs 82
Progress Graphs 86

VII Quizzes
Jean's Compassionate-Eating Quiz 30
Jean's Hypnotic-Responsiveness Quiz 75
Jean's Mindful-Eating Quiz 130
Jean's Social Support Quiz 190

Throughout the day I offer many prayers as the occasion arises:
"May you be healthy, and free from suffering."
"Just as I wish to be happy, may all beings be happy."
"May you enjoy vitality and ease of well-being."

I am not asking for everything to be better, or for all your dreams to
come true, but given that things are as they are and go as they go,
I wish for your well-being and happiness in the face of all the changing
circumstances. Things quite likely will not go ideally or according to
plan, so I wish for the growth of buoyancy, flexibility, and resiliency.
I wish for the nurturing of generosity and tolerance.

ED ESPE BROWN
TOMATO BLESSINGS AND RADISH TEACHINGS

PREFACE

The Impatient Dieter

Just start where you are.
PEMA CHÖDRÖN

If you want to get to a healthy, sustainable weight, you've got no choice but to start where you are. And yet if you could, you would choose to start elsewhere, wouldn't you? Given the choice, you would surely want to begin anywhere but right here, right now, just as you are. Whatever eating problem brought you to this book, you'd probably rather be:

- a good number of pounds lighter
- a dress size more like your shoe size than your age
- a peanut rather than apple-, pear-, or grapefruit-shaped

Given that you rarely, if ever, feel "light" or "thin" or "lean," it's easy to call yourself all kinds of mean, nasty names, to beat yourself up for letting yourself go, letting yourself get this fat, however fat "this fat" truly is.

The number on the scale isn't even the worst of it. How many veteran dieters step on the scale at their absolute heaviest? No, what's

worse is opening your eyes to a bright new day only to see the gloomy
shape of things:

- the bloat of your belly
- the girth of your thighs
- the spread of your hips

I understand, because for the longest time I wanted to be anywhere
but where you are. I would have tried just about anything that promised to control my appetite, curb my cravings, and shrink my fat cells.
I would have given just about anything to stop obsessing about what
I should and shouldn't eat, especially given how much I ate yesterday
and how little I believed I should eat . . . starting tomorrow.

Back in the 1970s, I invested in countless one-way tickets to thin. I
tried the Velveeta-and-salami diet, the white-food-only diet, the apple-
pie-for-breakfast diet, faux-chocolate diet shakes, diet pills with my diet
soda, juice fasts with my lemon water. (I drew the line at colon cleansing.) Desperately seeking thinner thighs in thirty days, a flat stomach in
no time flat, I also tried a range of punishing exercise regimens.

But the only return on my investment was a round-trip express
through momentarily slimmer that left me where I started, if not a
few pounds heavier and even more distraught. Sadly, three decades
later, the round-trip diet express is the same as it ever was—incredibly popular, largely ineffective, and surprisingly quick. I trust you've
climbed aboard more than once. Zipped back and forth between
weight loss and gain without ever stopping at weight maintenance.
Happily, I've found a far better, easier, and happier way to maintain a
healthy weight. But I'm getting ahead of myself.

If only there was a wise guide to intuitive slimness. Kind of like a GPS
that maps out the best weight-loss route according to your preferences;
that firmly redirects you when you get lost or encounter unforeseen

obstacles; that encourages you to learn from your mistakes rather than insulting you; that never gives up no matter how many wrong turns, impulsive decisions, and sudden stops you make. If only.

I had no choice but to become my own guide. Before I knew exactly where to go or how to get there, I did graduate studies in the school of hard knocks, my neighborhood figure salon. (That's what they called women's health clubs with shag carpeting.) When recurrent shin splints coerced me into a more sedentary line of work, I forged ahead as a syndicated fitness columnist until I realized that getting physical could only get you so far. Weight loss and other eating issues appeared to be as much about the mind as the body. ("Duh," you might say, but it wasn't that long ago that mind and body were viewed as good neighbors with good fences. Happily separate.) So I went back to school to explore the final frontier—the human mind.

Fast-forward twenty years, and my findings are striking: the smarter I got (the more mental slimming strategies I learned and taught clients), the thinner my clients got. Without dieting! The more I helped clients experience the dramatic, immediate difference a compassionate attitude makes (partially through cultivating my own self-compassion), the less they struggled in working toward their goals. The longer we worked together, the more weight they lost—10, 20, 30, 50, 100 pounds. Many got happily slimmer, which is not to say they all lived slimly ever after.

You need read no further than the end of this sentence to learn the most valuable lesson of my two decades as a therapist specializing in eating issues, and the most important point of this guidebook: *Getting a handle on eating issues is a journey, not the jaunt American dieters are determined to make it.*

That journey is incredibly personal. I now know there's no such thing as THE best route, because the best route for you may not be so great for your binge-eating neighbor, your yo-yo dieting cousin, your carb-loving sister. There are surely more and less direct routes to healthy slimness, but there are only a handful of psychological routes worth traveling.

This is a guidebook for your weight-loss journey from a guide who has traveled the distance from impatient dieter to compassionate-eating guide. Inside you will discover attitude- and shape-altering suggestions based on cutting-edge research from three separate but related schools of thought—cognitive-behavioral therapy, hypnotherapy, and meditation; from four scientifically proven routes for anyone interested in eating with more control and less compulsion: self-compassion, positive suggestion, conscious awareness, and social support; and from four sets of guided practices, the very same practices that have helped my clients.

Follow in my clients' footsteps, and you'll learn how to:

- cultivate self-compassion and get a handle on emotional eating
- give yourself positive suggestions and lose twice as much weight and keep it off longer—long enough to establish healthy eating habits
- binge less by eating more mindfully
- stay the weight-loss course with in-person or online help

My clients' transformative experiences on the first route you'll explore, self-compassion, have changed the way I guide clients along the other three routes of hypnosis, mindfulness, and group support. More than simply a route, self-compassion, or consciously cultivating a compassionate attitude toward oneself, is the guiding principle of this book and what makes the weight-loss journey possible. Self-compassion is the missing ingredient in every diet and weight-loss strategy. It has the power to turn mistakes into learning experiences, and transform gloomy failures into bright new possibilities.

The wow power of self-compassion has not only transformed my work, it's indelibly changed me. I had almost abandoned my life's dream of getting a book published when I met Chris Germer, a remarkably kind psychologist and big proponent of self-compassion practice. We started talking, and shortly thereafter I began practicing the first self-compassion practice you will learn—*metta,* also known as loving-kindness meditation. Not to lose weight, mind you. Weight maintenance had become second nature decades earlier. No, I put myself on the metta diet in the Latin sense of the word—*diaeta*—as a way of breathing, eating, and living. The results astonished me. I quickly felt calmer, happier, and more appreciative of the people in my life. And suddenly, or so it seemed, a book began to take shape.

The title may be *The Self-Compassion Diet,* but what you won't find in these pages is a traditional American "diet." This book contains no forbidden food lists, no suggested portion sizes, no calorie-cutting strategies. If you want to lose weight and regain more, traditional diets reliably deliver. You deserve more—a more harmonious relationship with food, a more sustainable weight-loss strategy. Given all the weight-loss plans you have under your belt or elasticized waistband, these less-traveled psychotherapeutic routes I am about to describe may sound more like dead ends. I encourage a healthy mix of skepticism and curiosity, especially when assessing a new weight-loss strategy. Trust is built over time and with experience, and we've only just met.

But follow along, and what you *will* find is that this no-diet diet delivers far more than any promises made by diet pills, drinks, or other weight-loss products without the long list of negative side effects. In addition to intuitive slimness, this eat-all-you-can-comfortably-eat plan predictably provides an incredible array of physical, mental, and emotional health benefits, including decreased risk of heart disease, diabetes, and other life-threatening illnesses; increased concentration, perspective, and hope; lower levels of stress, anxiety, and depression, and greater connection with loved ones.

I'm excited about helping you to get slim without the deprivation and self-loathing associated with dieting. Like I said, this simple plan provides flexibility within structure, but no structured food plan. If you insist on sticking to a diet, even if you're considering or have undergone gastric bypass surgery, you can still benefit from this book. But I urge you to consider taking a break from counting points, calories, or fat grams while you explore this exciting new terrain.

Ideally, you will be so enthralled by *The Self-Compassion Diet,* you will explore all four weight-loss routes. But if you go directly to the route(s) that most excite you, you will do just as well. Just as there's no best way to lose weight, there's no best way to read this book. I'll show you the road map, but you will definitely want to honor your preferences in charting the course. This is your guidebook for your real-life weight-loss journey. Read it, write in it, dog-ear the pages, keep it bed-side, travel with it, reread it. *The Self-Compassion Diet* is all about finding *your* way. If you proceed with self-compassion, you will find it.

INTRODUCTION

Planning Your Journey

*I don't think it takes more time to be
mindful than it takes to be mindless.*

MYLA KABAT-ZINN

You've got a clear destination—intuitive slimness—but only a vague sense of how to get there from here, especially if you've never tried bypassing that old bridge to weight gain: dieting. If you're thinking you could use an accurate road map right about now, I think you're right. But you've already got one; you're holding it in your hands. At first glance, this program looks a little different than other weight-loss maps. It is. The big difference: there's more than one way to travel through it. *The Self-Compassion Diet* lays out four separate weight-loss routes: (1) the path of self-compassion, often called loving-kindness; (2) the path of hypnosis, sometimes referred to as positive suggestion; (3) the path of mindfulness, also known as conscious awareness; and (4) the path of social support, used interchangeably in these pages with the term "compassionate community."

If you were expecting one direct route to your desired weight, this multi-route approach may seem confusing. And if choice frequently makes your head spin or your eyes glaze over, take my hand. As your compassionate-eating guide, my job is to show you around, point out the best ways to go. So sit back, relax, and let me help you plan a comfortable, customized trip. But first, let me show you the lay of the land, the layout of the book.

The four weight-loss routes covered in *The Self-Compassion Diet* are spread out over nine different chapters, two chapters per route, plus one chapter on where to go once you have integrated the practices into your life. The first chapter for each route gives you the theory behind the guided practices in the companion chapter that follows it. If you want a comprehensive view of the routes—a readable review of key concepts, theoretical perspectives, historical events, and landmark studies, plus inspiring cases (my clients' and my own)—you can go straight to chapters 1, 3, 5, and 7. If you'd like to work with the practices—traditional meditations, guided visualizations, hypnotic trances, and writing exercises—turn to chapters 2, 4, 6, and 8. If you need guidance for the next leg of your journey—for how to discover your most effective practices and find supportive travel mates—continue to chapter 9.

For a fuller view of the whole compassion-enhancing landscape, take a look at the following chapter previews: Chapter 1 explains self-compassion, and how a little goes a long way toward sustainable weight loss. Chapter 2 demonstrates what a measurable difference self-compassion makes by assessing how self-compassionate you are before and after the six guided practices that are provided in the chapter. Chapter 3 explains why the age-old technique of hypnosis helps you lose more weight and keep it off longer, long enough to establish healthy eating habits. Chapter 4 poses twenty-one questions to help you assess your hypnotic ability, and then, according to your ability, shows you how to hypnotize yourself slim with six winning suggestions. Chapter 5 explains why eating with awareness helps you gain control and lose weight by connecting the disparate dots between the ancient awareness practices of mindfulness meditation and the modern-day wisdom from food science. Chapter 6 shows you how to have your cake, mindfully eat it, and lose weight too, with one mindful-eating assessment and eight guided visualizations and eating meditations. Chapter 7 explains why recruiting the support of at least one successful weight-loss partner, or perhaps more, helps you achieve lasting success. Chapter 8 helps you further understand and make use of your current support network before guiding you through six illuminating practices for building a stronger network. Chapter 9 helps you organize your old weight-loss toolkit, and offers final suggestions for choosing and committing to favorite practices for your continuing journey.

So you can see, the odd chapters are theoretical, the even are practical. Except for chapter 9, which thinks it's even. In addition to the twenty-six guided practices in the first eight chapters, you get four practical suggestions in the ninth and final chapter. All the chapters have one thing in common: sidebars. You know, those boxed features in magazines and books. Whether the chapter is odd or even, you can count on "Finding Thinspiration," beacons of hope and motivation where you least expect them: eating in, watching TV, dining out. You'll also learn to trust your food-scientist alter ego with "Personal Slimming Lessons," experiments that help you challenge common dieting wisdom. What's more, you'll find ample opportunity to cultivate a kinder, gentler attitude with "Think Kind Self-Thoughts," caring responses to your harshest self-criticisms. Plus, smart answers to FAQs (Frequently Asked Questions) or, as I like to call them, NSQs (No Stupid Questions).

Still with me? Good, because the plan's about to get even simpler. Forget about keeping track of the number of chapters and practices, and remember this: you've basically got four ways to go through this book, and no wrong ways.

Option One: The first option is the simplest way to go. Read this book cover to cover. Read it without practicing; even a simple

read-through of *The Self-Compassion Diet* will make you smarter, if
not a little kinder. Perusing these pages with intellectual curiosity, you
will become more knowledgeable about the psychological approaches
to sustainable weight loss. Page by page, you will come to view yourself with more loving-kindness. And if you're contemplating weight
loss, but aren't ready to spring into action, the act of reading will help
you get ready.

Option Two: For the most comprehensive approach to the book,
read *and* practice from cover to cover. It's a tall and maybe impractical order, but it's my very best suggestion. Route by route, learn the
theory, then try the practices. Start with self-compassion: work fifteen
to twenty minutes of your favorite self-compassion, mindfulness, or
hypnosis practice into your daily routine, and find the support of others when you are ready. The initial time investment is a little steep; if
you tried a practice a day, it would take a month to try them all. But
the dividends of loving-kindness, unconscious wisdom, conscious
awareness, and positive support are invaluable, and they start paying
off immediately.

Option Three: If you're crazy busy or busy enough, the third
option is a time-saver and allows for two ways in one. (1) If you're
clearly done with dieting and you've already chosen one particular
route, go directly to the theory and practice of your chosen route.
Read the theory, do the practices. The practices are self-explanatory,
so you could theoretically skip the theory. But in the rush to practice, some important things, such as clarity and inspiration, might
get lost. (2) If you have yet to choose your best route(s), check out
your options. Learn about the four routes in chapters 1, 3, 5, and 7;
notice which appeal; and then turn to the most appealing companion
chapter and try the practices. For example, if chapter 3 invites you to
try hypnosis, advance to the trance practices in the next chapter. Even
if hypnosis holds little allure, I encourage you to visit chapter 4 for

the cognitive-behavioral therapy (CBT) exercises, which help revamp counterproductive thoughts and behaviors. These CBT exercises help you do more than accomplish basic weight-loss tasks (setting goals, identifying eating patterns, and charting your progress)—they help you snap to attention and jump-start weight loss.

Option Four: If you want to get the feel of *The Self-Compassion Diet* without reading the whole book, the fourth option gives you the bare minimum and a perceptible preview of the enormous benefits that come with time and practice. Read chapter 1, skipping over the sidebars, and proceed to chapter 2. Take the Compassionate-Eating Quiz and find out how self-compassionate you are. Do the first and simplest practice: Loving-Kindness Meditation. If you have got the time and inclination, do two more: Compassionate Advisor and Head-to-Toe Appreciation. If the fourth option leaves you wanting more, reconsider options one through three.

The self-compassionate diet succeeds where others fail because, among other reasons, it encourages you to find the way that works best *for you.* If you can't imagine taking a break from traditional dieting as I've suggested, then follow your diet plan and *The Self-Compassion Diet.* The combination will enhance your chances of success. I know it sounds counterintuitive—be softer on yourself, lose more weight—but it works. If giving yourself a hard time worked better, I suspect you would be reading a boot-camp diet book right now.

That said, in at least two cases, what works best is neither obvious nor intuitive. If you have a history of trauma or a life-threatening eating disorder, don't try these practices alone. Enlist the help of a trusted therapist or another health-care professional. If you've got medical concerns, including issues related to gastric bypass surgery, consult your physician before starting this or any eating program. If you're the picture of health, you will still want to prepare yourself. To help you get ready, set, and practice, consider the following suggestions:

GET READY: If you just want to read the book cover to cover, find yourself a quiet moment, a comfortable chair, and a good reading lamp, and you're all set. But if you're keen on practicing too, success comes more easily when you make time and space for regular practice. Any amount of time you can set aside for practice is good, but fifteen to twenty minutes a day is ideal. If twenty minutes seems like an eternity or impossibility, consider doing several shorter sessions throughout the day. If a quarter of an hour feels like a warm-up, beef up your practice to thirty minutes or an hour by adding periods of silence or continuing with the basic elements of the practice. While there's no best time to practice, there's something to be said for practicing at or around the same time of day. That way, rather than thinking about when to practice, you're in the habit of just doing it.

GET SET: A space conducive to the self-compassion practices is one that's safe and quiet, away from distractions—the phone and significant others, pets included. (Unless Fluffy or Fido is especially well-behaved.) Some practitioners find lighting incense or candles enhances the quietude of the space. Feel free to experiment with the setting and the seating. Most of the practices in this book can be done sitting or lying down, except for the writing and eating practices. Those are easier to do sitting at a table or near another flat surface. A meditation cushion may be the traditional seating arrangement for the mindfulness and self-compassion practices, but it is by no means essential. If you'd rather spend time in an MRI machine than on a *zafu,* a Japanese sitting cushion, try a recliner, a couch, or a chaise lounge. And if back pain or another medical condition makes sitting or lying for any length of time uncomfortable, you can always do these practices standing.

If you notice preventable distractions, address them before you begin practicing rather than hoping that they won't bother you. Of course, you can't prevent all distractions. Between your outer world (barking dogs, sirens) and inner experience (physical, emotional, and mental reactions), it's only a matter of time before your attention is divided, diverted, or otherwise disturbed. If you are unable to remove all your surrounding distractions, think of them as party guests: it's then easier to acknowledge them and maintain focus. Some guests leave promptly; others overstay their welcome. Rather than showing unwanted guests the door, your job as the gracious host is to stay with them, even the high-maintenance ones, for the duration.

PRACTICE: For a clear sense of the intention behind a practice, read the introduction, then follow the script as written. If it's a short practice, you can read through the script once or twice, close your eyes if you like, and mentally guide yourself through it. For the longer practices, you will need to keep your eyes open and meditate on the words as well as the suggested images, ideas, and feelings. If with faithful practice, you come to know the longer scripts by heart, you've got a choice: eyes open or closed. For a deeper, more relaxing experience, especially with the guided visualizations and hypnotic trances, consider enlisting an actual or virtual guide—a generous friend to read you the practice scripts, or a recording device that can play your reading voice. For a best-of-both-worlds approach, you might try listening to *The Self-Compassion Diet* audio program. At the touch of a button, my voice will virtually guide you through many of the practices contained in these pages.

Most of the practices begin by inviting you to focus on the breath, and settle into a comfortable breathing rhythm. There's nothing more natural than breathing, but conscious breathing is easier said than done. Rest assured—a clear understanding of the instructions and regular practice definitely makes it easier. "Focus on the breath" simply means direct your attention to the rise and fall of your chest, the air at the entrance of your nostrils, the sound of the breath in your ears . . . any aspect of your breathing that's easy to observe. When the mind naturally wanders from your focus, the task becomes refocusing over and over again. "Settling into a comfortable breathing rhythm" calls for letting the inhalation naturally deepen, the exhalation gradually lengthen. Nothing more. And yet, many practitioners try to force the issue by inhaling a big gulp of air or exhaling a huge sigh. Like restful sleep, you can't force deep breathing. If you find yourself forcibly trying, then pause, refocus, and practice patience. The breath will naturally settle into comfort. When you've finished practicing, keep breathing as you reorient yourself to your surroundings and reflect on your experience.

Once you've tried a practice, feel free to tailor it to your strengths and interests. If visualizing is a turnoff and writing a turn-on, for example, turn the guided visualizations into journal-writing exercises. The most effective practices are the ones that are beneficial and doable—the ones that find a place in your daily routine. They aren't the ones that you think you should do, but won't do.

You can always make more preparations, but if you're serious about getting to a healthy, sustainable weight, you will want to stop preparing and start practicing. Preparing is an important step forward, but it can't get you where you're going. Ditto for know-how. All the know-how in the world can only take you so far. Transforming your eating habits also takes calm, conscious awareness and loving-kindness, all of which take practice. It's easy to buy a book or a CD, try on a new idea, make a temporary change. But lasting transformation—well, that takes practice.

PART I

Self-Compassion

The Power of Loving-Kindness

THE KINDER, GENTLER THERAPIST

Often we can achieve an even better result when we stumble yet are willing to start over, when we don't give up after a mistake, when something doesn't come easily but we throw ourselves into trying, when we're not afraid to appear less than perfectly polished.

SHARON SALZBERG

From my blue leather easy-chair, I watch psychotherapy clients shrink before my eyes. You might joke, as many do, that I shrink people for a living. But to be fair, my clients have been shrinking themselves under my watch through my career's many incarnations. Listening to countless stories of pounds lost and regained these last three decades, I never would have guessed that more self-compassion, not self-discipline, is the answer to dieters' prayers. I never could have predicted that a more forgiving attitude toward oneself and others would help those desperately seeking a slim physique to have a happier, easier, if not speedier time with losing weight.

As soon as clients tap into the power of self-compassion, out goes the "battle" from the battle of the bulge. When they take a kinder, gentler view of their bodies, their whole selves, as well as a softer stance toward their imperfect food choices and daily weight fluctuations, they struggle less and eat more healthfully almost immediately.

As soon as my clients hear the word "self-compassion," a tenet of Eastern philosophy that is just making inroads in Western psychology, clients start visibly changing: their eyes brighten, their expressions soften, their shoulders relax. It's as if they have been starving for this softer stance toward their shape, a more accepting, less competitive attitude toward weight loss that has nothing to do with deprivation and self-loathing, and everything to do with nurturance and self-acceptance. They get a taste of self-compassion, and suddenly they're hungry for more.

Q Can self-compassion curb emotional eating?

A Apparently so. Researchers and therapists have found that a modest dose of self-compassion prevents the self-criticism and negative feelings that can fuel overeating. Just remembering that everyone eats junk food sometimes and that a lapse doesn't constitute a disastrous relapse, study subjects ate with restraint after falling off the (diet) wagon.

COMPASSION TASTE TEST

It's subtle, so you may not realize that you got a taste of compassion as soon as you started reading this book. To get a better sense of what I'm talking about, take a moment right now and focus on the word "self-compassion" and notice the subtle shifts in your mood, your posture. Even better, imagine a compassionate friend, a dear person or pet, gazing at you with loving eyes, and observe the feelings, bodily sensations, thoughts, and images that arise.

Very different, isn't it, than your visceral reaction to words typically associated with weight loss? Think "diet," "exercise regimen," "self-discipline," and again notice shifts in your attitude, your sense of well-being, the tension in your body. Are the corners of your mouth curling up or frown-ward? Tell yourself for the umpteenth time how you really ought to start losing weight today and see what happens to your mood. Better yet, imagine Dr. Phil's fist pump on the cover of *The Ultimate Weight Solution* or just picture a powerful fist urging *you*, insisting that *you* stop making excuses and start shaping up pronto. How do you feel now?

Clearly, self-compassion tastes nothing like self-discipline. But how does self-compassion facilitate weight loss? Wouldn't self-compassion make you softer on yourself, more self-indulgent? Isn't self-discipline the only way to go? Ah yes, self-discipline. That's what new clients expect me to magically conjure up in order to counteract cravings for ice cream, cookies, or, in Katherine's case, candy bars. Never in this proud grandmother's wildest dreams did she imagine that self-compassion would be the antidote to her Snickers addiction. Instead of comforting herself with that creamy, nutty goodness, Katherine found she could soothe herself and stay the weight-loss course by practicing loving-kindness meditation.

I begin with Katherine's story because her weight-loss history is every dieter's, and because she was one of the first on my caseload to harness the power of self-compassion. Plus, she's a hoot! "I'm seventy-one years old and I'm not dead yet," Katherine announced in our first session. This no-nonsense gal with L. L. Bean fashion sense and kind blue eyes had "tried everything"—diets, diet pills, weight-loss groups at work, yet "nothing worked" . . . for long. Determined to go snorkeling with her grandchildren, this grandmother was willing to explore weight-loss roads less traveled if she could drop a few skirt sizes and feel comfortable in fins and a snorkel mask.

Katherine traveled the four routes mapped out in these pages. She kept a food log, a tried-and-true cognitive-behavioral technique; she listened to self-hypnosis audio CDs; she savored meals at a café table bought for the sole purpose of mindful eating, and every day she cultivated self-compassion. Happily, steadily, and without depriving herself of the occasional Hershey's Kiss, she lost fifteen pounds in twelve weeks. (Dieters often fantasize about rapid results, but, like Katherine's, a healthy, self-compassionate weight-loss rate is no more than one to two pounds a week.) More than any one technique, it was her attitude that allowed Katherine to ultimately succeed. "It [this

approach] worked" because dietary transgressions were no longer pro-
nouncements on her weak will or predictions of certain failure. With a
kinder, more accepting attitude toward herself, what were once "transgressions" became invitations to review her missteps, remember her
intentions, and recommit herself to paying attention. What thrilled
Katherine as much, if not more, than losing the weight and fitting back
into a favorite Burberry skirt was what she gained: compassion for
herself and her three daughters. "I don't have to be perfect," she said,
eyes bright with delight. "I'm more forgiving of myself and my girls."

PERSONAL SLIMMING LESSON

Chew On This

If you want to lose weight, you should chew each bite 20-40 times—at least, that's
what some mindful-eating authorities say. As a weight-loss strategy, is chewing your
food a set number of times effective? Sustainable? Compassionate? To help you find
perspective and answers, here's a short history lesson and a little experiment.

First the history lesson: Chewing as a slimming strategy was first introduced
more than a century ago by a self-proclaimed diet expert named Horace
Fletcher. Fletcher, also known as "The Great Masticator," developed quite the
following—Henry James, Upton Sinclair, John D. Rockefeller, among other
Victorian-era glitterati. If you follow Fletcher's advice—chew every bite 32 times or
100 times per minute—you'll probably drop a few pounds.

But is counting chews for you? Try this little experiment: At the next meal, make it
a point to chew each bite at least 20 times. No matter how chewy the entrée, chew,
chew, chew, and observe. Does robotic chewing help you eat more mindfully? Does
mashing each bite to a smooth paste enhance or detract from your dining pleasure?
How does it affect your jaw during and after the meal? Can you imagine counting
chews for a day, a week, a lifetime? If you can, keep counting. If not, you never
have to count another bite.

THE BUDDHA'S PROMISE

When I was an impatient dieter three-plus decades ago, if someone
had told me about self-compassion as a weight-loss strategy, I would

have thought they had joined a cult or a New Age therapy group. Lose weight without dieting? Go on! Two decades later, I was more receptive, thanks in large part to Jon Kabat-Zinn and other dedicated meditators who introduced ancient mindfulness practices to the modern medical establishment and the public at large. I was still skeptical, I realized, when I attended a workshop on loving-kindness meditation, also known as metta meditation. How could meditating on loving feelings effect positive change?

As the radiant, serene, beloved meditation instructor expounded on the widespread benefits of this compassion-enhancing meditation, my skepticism wrestled with my curiosity. This petite blonde with the beatific expression seemed to embody the most apparent benefits that the Buddha had promised way back when—facial radiance, mental serenity, eternal belovedness. Surely the instructor was born with a sunny disposition, I thought. Surely the Buddha's promise was too good to be true.

Turns out the Buddha was on to something. As I have gotten to know colleagues who practice metta, as I have sat in awe in front of my incredibly shrinking clients, as I have read up on the exciting new research on self-compassion, my thinking has slowly but surely changed. Self-compassion, I am now convinced, is transformative. Self-compassion (it's worth repeating) is the missing ingredient in every diet and most other weight-loss strategies. Self-compassion practices are recipes for all manner of personal change. If Oprah ate more compassionately, there's no guarantee she would never backslide again. But losing weight without self-compassion is an uphill battle, pretty much a losing battle at that.

COMPASSION 101

What is this thing called self-compassion? If compassion, as the *American Heritage Dictionary* defines it, is "a deep awareness of the suffering of another coupled with the wish to relieve it," then

self-compassion is a deep awareness of *one's own* suffering, coupled
with the very same wish. More instructive perhaps is the definition
developed by Kristin Neff, the University of Texas professor who created the self-compassion scale used in psychology research today.[1]
Self-compassion, according to Neff, is comprised of three essential
components: *mindful awareness, self-kindness, and common humanity.*

Self-compassion starts with mindful awareness and the judgment-
free perspective that comes with it. Mindful awareness or mindfulness
is simply giving your full attention to the present moment with as little
judgment or as much acceptance as you can muster. Mindfulness calls
for sitting with your suffering and simply noticing it, instead of getting emotionally entangled in it or, conversely, ignoring or avoiding
it. In other words, it involves wading into painful feelings as opposed
to drowning in or swimming from them. Self-kindness is what it
sounds like: treating yourself with care and understanding rather
than beating yourself up with harsh criticisms. The understanding
that suffering is part of the human experience, that you are not alone
and others suffer similarly, is the essence of common humanity.

For veteran dieters, self-compassion means never having to promise you'll be "good" starting Monday. If you are a compassionate
eater, you dispense with the promises and hang out with whatever
uncomfortable feelings arise after one too many indulgent spoonfuls.
You befriend emotional and physical discomfort and treat it like a
welcome houseguest, not a housefly. Yes, sometimes you make less
than healthful choices. People make mistakes. You don't take solace
in unwholesome comparisons, like "At least I'm not as fat as that fat
actress!" Not when you feel a kinship with the great, multigenera-
tional sorority that, on occasion, seeks refuge in the refrigerator.

If you are a compassionate eater, the only promise worth making is
the one ex-smokers make: to learn from mistakes. Rather than person-
ify that old definition of insanity—continuing to do the same thing

and expecting different results—you look for lessons from indul-
gences. "What can I learn?" is a far more compassionate question than
the one that dieters typically ask: "How can I lose ten pounds fast?"
The latter question leaves little room for mindful awareness, self-
kindness, and common humanity. In the outer quest for the magic
weight-loss cure, there's really no point in cultivating inner awareness.
The "lose weight fast" question is a self-critical one; it presupposes
the questioner is unattractive, and therefore unacceptable at his or
her present weight. In this desperate mind-set, it's not only out of
the question to feel a kinship with other overeaters, it's unbearable.
It suddenly seems so right to seek comfort in unwholesome comparisons with anyone screwing up more royally—your nosy neighbor,
gossipy aunt, overbearing book-club president—anyone who makes
you feel comparatively thin. Not that you seek out the company of
those you consider "royal screwups." After all, facing your weight fears
is uncomfortable. But when you're bloated with self-contempt, there's
carb-free comfort in the realization: "At least you haven't ballooned
like so-and-so!"

Self-compassion is a personality trait, like optimism or extrover-
sion, but it's also a trainable mental skill with big benefits. According
to numerous psychological studies, research subjects who entertained
self-compassionate thoughts experienced greater emotional resiliency and psychological well-being. They were measurably happier,
wiser, more capable, and curious. They felt greater life satisfaction
and social connectedness, and they took more personal initiative and
responsibility. On the flip side, they were generally less depressed and
anxious. They ruminated less, thought fewer self-critical thoughts,
and were less afraid of failure.

Most researchers have measured the difference that self-compassion makes in a single day, but Kristin Neff, the one researcher
who tracked subjects for an entire month, found that ongoing

self-compassion training worked like antidepressants without the side effects. It bolstered subjects' positive emotional mind-sets and weakened their negative mental states for the duration of the study.[2] For a closer look at a mind meditating on pure compassion, a group of University of Wisconsin neuroscientists conducted brain-imaging studies of Buddhist monks meditating on loving-kindness. How they found thirty-two volunteers willing to meditate in the claustrophobic confines of MRI machines is hard to fathom, but that they did. Compassion, it turns out, is literally mind-altering! Not only does cultivating an attitude of loving-kindness stimulate the parts of the brain associated with empathy and maternal love (the insula and the temporal parietal junction) in men and women, it promises to dampen activity in the brain areas associated with depression and anxiety.[3]

Self-compassion offers many of the benefits of its cousin self-esteem (the perception of self-worth) without the downside. Trying to bolster self-esteem can inadvertently encourage narcissistic thoughts and discourage accurate self-evaluation. When you're running low on self-esteem, it's certainly easier to hide personal shortcomings than to acknowledge them. And compared to sitting with the discomfort of low self-esteem, it can be much more comfortable, if not enjoyable, to put down anyone, who, by comparison, makes you look a whole lot better. Sure, it can be lonely at the top, but that's the price many are willing to pay for the temporary high of self-esteem. Because it can fluctuate like the stock market, it's hard to depend on self-esteem when you screw up or otherwise really need it. And it's extremely difficult to boost.

Self-compassion, on the other hand, is never in short supply, even when demand is high and self-esteem low. Whether you're down on your luck or blessed with good fortune and enviable traits, self-compassion is always accessible. And unifying. The emphasis on common humanity—that the human race is one big not-always-so-happy family—encourages more accurate self-appraisals and a greater feeling of interconnectedness. What's more, unlike self-esteem, self-compassion can be cultivated.[4] The reason why you can more easily boost self-compassion than self-esteem is unclear, but when you think about it, kindly acknowledging personal limitations sounds much more doable than spinning negative self-evaluations into positive ones.

AN ENCOURAGING STUDY

The study that confirmed my long-held beliefs and pushed me to finally write this book was the investigation of whether cultivating self-compassion could curb emotional overeating in veteran dieters. Promoting self-compassionate attitudes toward eating was the subject of an exciting 2007 study conducted by Wake Forest University psychologists.[5] Some study subjects were instructed to eat a "forbidden food" (a donut) and then taste a variety of candies while watching TV, an activity strongly linked with emotional eating. About half were prompted to think compassionate thoughts between the donut and the candy. The prompted half was reminded that everyone eats unhealthfully sometimes, and eating one donut was no reason to feel bad about yourself. The other half went straight from the first to the second course.

The results defied researchers' expectations: dieting subjects who entertained compassionate thoughts sampled the candies, but did not gobble them up. By simply remembering that everyone eats junk food sometimes, that a lapse doesn't constitute a full-blown relapse, these college coeds ate with restraint after falling off the (diet) wagon, much like nondieters in previous studies. A modest dose of self-compassion seemed to prevent the self-criticism and negative feelings that can fuel overeating. Not so for the subjects who got no encouragement to reflect on self-compassion. The dieters who weren't prompted to think kindly of themselves ate significantly more candy then their kinder counterparts.

What didn't happen was equally noteworthy: cultivating self-compassion *did not* lead to self-indulgence or self-pity. Rather, it seemed to help dieters maintain perspective, take more personal responsibility, and inhibit their candy consumption.

Breaking the vicious, paradoxical cycle of rigid dieting and overeating may require nothing more than establishing a friendlier paradox: take charge of your eating by letting go of rigid dietary control and by reacting to "diet failures" more gently. Easier said than done, I know. Stuffing unhappy feelings about such "failures" with more food can be comfortably familiar, momentarily relieving. And yet, the researchers' conclusion is worth restating, underscoring, if not mounting in a magnetic fridge frame: a spoonful of self-compassion makes it possible to have a bowl of ice cream without polishing off the whole pint. A steady, compassion-rich diet makes it downright doable to cope with whatever life serves you without a calorie free-for-all.

> **THINK SELF-KIND THOUGHTS**
>
> **Your Inner Critic:**
>   I can't believe I ate _____
>   *(fill in a recent overindulgence).*
>   I'm such a _____ *(something mean and nasty you call yourself).*
>
> **Your Compassionate Response:**
>   _____
>   _____
>   _____
>   _____

These findings support existing arguments that strict dieting can lead to overeating. In assessing effective obesity treatments, a group of Medicare researchers recently reviewed the range of dieting studies and determined that diets, in the long run, *don't* work.[6] The researchers' conclusions challenge the popular belief that diets lead to lasting weight loss. Diets, they found, contribute more to weight gain than loss, thereby increasing the very health risks they aim to decrease. It's cruel but statistically true; no matter how much weight dieters lose, they commonly regain more.

When you view, through the kind eyes of compassion scholars, the cruel truth that dieting statistically contributes more to weight gain than loss, it suddenly makes perfect sense why the tedious math problems that so many diet doctors do are counterproductive. You know the algebraic equations I'm talking about: if a couch potato consumes this many chips daily, watches that many hours of TV nightly, how many pounds will he pack on by New Year's Day? Diet-doctor logic proves illogical because it is distressing. It inspires people to become couch potatoes who bury their heads in more chips in an act of decreased self-awareness, or what psychologists call "cognitive narrowing." In the face of such grim inevitabilities, dejected dieters often narrow their focus to the immediate pleasure of a favorite snack. I trust you are familiar with the fleeting pleasure of cognitive narrowing.

A HARD SELL

Self-compassion, I'm well aware, is a hard a sell in our quick-fix, diet-crazed society. The evidence in favor of self-compassion is sparse. To date, there's only the one published study on eating problems and self-compassion. A team of British researchers has conducted a promising study on compassion training for bulimics.[7] And a doctoral student established a positive link between self-compassion and exercise motivation.[8] But neither has yet published their findings.

With self-compassion, weight loss will never be as quick as it is with the crash diet du jour. Dieters who insist on dramatic results yesterday aren't all that interested in being kind to themselves today, not if it's possible to fit into a smaller pair of jeans by next weekend. Bring on the tasteless frozen entrees, the thimble-sized portions, the endless caloric equations. Waist watchers keep salivating like Pavlovian dogs for the next big diet because there's never a shortage of reasons to lose weight now: a reunion, a wedding, a new bikini, a potential beau—and because, as bestselling anti-diet book writer Geneen Roth says, for every diet there is an equal and opposite binge. There's always more weight to lose.

America's breathless pace of living also makes self-compassion a hard sell. Despite the mounting scientific evidence on the far-reaching health benefits of meditation, despite bestselling books like Elizabeth Gilbert's *Eat, Pray, Love,* despite Oprah's endorsements of spiritually enlightened ideas à la Eckhart Tolle, meditating on loving-kindness is still considered a snooze by many. Ours is a fast-paced society that values "doing" more than "being," exhaustion more than rest, punishing discipline more than loving-kindness. People tend to think that unless you are willing to sit on a meditation cushion in an Indian ashram at the feet of a teacher with an unpronounceable name for several lifetimes, you can forget about reaping the benefits. Or so goes the thinking.

Those who could most use a compassionate attitude toward themselves—often dieting women and teenagers—are naturally inclined toward self-criticism. Women are born and bred to be compassionate; at least, that's the stereotype. But it appears they are also hardwired to be self-critical and ruminative, suggesting they may actually be the less self-compassionate sex, especially during the tumultuous teens. This is not to say that teenaged boys are full of kindness for themselves as they pass through this hormonal rite of passage. No, adolescence, with all its heavy-duty self-evaluation and social comparison, is a self-compassion low point across the board. But given that unflattering self-evaluations and comparisons tend to fuel eating problems, this little-known feminine tendency to get mired in unkind thought may help explain why fat and other food preoccupations are enduring feminist issues.

I may be closer to senility than puberty, but I haven't forgotten how to dwell on my shortcomings and feel adolescent angst. I could criticize myself for failing to help the client who really needed self-compassion training, but instead chose an intestinal cleanse. "Intellectually, I know I *should* be compassionate," Bella explained on the way out the door, "but I don't really know what it means to be nice to myself." I could definitely beat myself up for letting her walk, but in my heart, I know she wasn't ready for such an unconventional, all-encompassing approach to permanent weight loss. She was still holding out hope for the next quick fix.

FINDING THINSPIRATION

Clip 'n' Save

If you've ever had your eye on the dieter's prize—rapid weight loss—you know it's easy to lose sight of the long-term goal. Nope, I'm not talking about losing another ten pounds or squeezing into smaller jeans, but achieving a healthier relationship with food. You know, eating normally. To help you reset your sights on this more realistic and hopeful goal, I've dug out my favorite definition of normal eating by nutritionist Ellyn Satter from Madison, Wisconsin. It's definitely worth clipping 'n' saving:

"Normal eating is going to the table hungry and eating until you are satisfied. It is being able to choose food you like and eat it and truly get enough of it—not just stop eating because you think you should. Normal eating is being able to give some thought to your food selection so you get nutritious food, but not being so wary and restrictive that you miss out on enjoyable food. Normal eating is giving yourself permission to eat sometimes because you are happy, sad, or bored, or just because it feels good. Normal eating is mostly three meals a day, or four or five, or it can be choosing to munch along the way. It is leaving some cookies on the plate because you know you can have some again tomorrow, or it is eating more now because they taste so wonderful. Normal eating is overeating at times, feeling stuffed and uncomfortable. And it can be under-eating at times and wishing you had more. Normal eating is trusting your body to make up for your mistakes in eating. Normal eating takes up some of your time and attention, but keeps its place as only one important area of your life. In short, normal eating is flexible. It varies in response to your hunger, your schedule, your proximity to food, and your feelings."[9]

AN INFORMAL EXPERIMENT

Mind you, I wasn't completely sold on the power of self-compassion until I conducted my own informal experiments, instead of merely observing my clients. Betty, a fifty-year-old psychotherapy client and horseback-riding instructor with a freckled face and teenage giggle, may have been my best student and teacher. This active mother of two had made strides exploring the terrain of mindfulness: she had lost 10 pounds and gotten a grip on her anxiety, but she wanted more (a "beltable" waistline) and less (30 pounds less). She desperately wanted to get rid of her muffin-top, she told me more than once, each time squeezing a handful of belly fat for emphasis. Despite her active lifestyle and ten-pound weight loss, she felt incapable of losing weight. With little to lose and much to gain, I shared my passion for self-compassion.

Once Betty understood that I wasn't talking about positive thinking, that she didn't risk becoming jarringly optimistic, she was eager to learn more. She went online and assessed her current level of self-compassion,[10] and researched the core concepts of mindful awareness, self-kindness, and common humanity. Betty liked the ideas of self-kindness and mindful awareness, but bristled at the concept of common humanity. Feeling a kinship with "dumpy housewives" everywhere, she admitted with some embarrassment, might destine her to be "dumpy" like them. She was willing, however, to send loving-kindness to select apple-shaped acquaintances, and then report back.

The results were dramatic and immediate. After a number of traditional meditations and guided visualizations, Betty showed up with a softer hairstyle and a sunnier expression. A few weeks later, she sashayed into my office wearing more flattering, comfortable jeans—one size smaller. She stopped weighing herself (the scale hadn't been much of a friend), so she wasn't sure how much weight she had lost. But judging from all the compliments she got two months into the training, it was a noticeable amount.

Echoing Katherine's sentiments, the qualitative life changes Betty made were as important, if not more so, than the quantitative. "I'm gardening, horseback riding, doing what I love," she reported, "and I feel zero self-criticism about my body!" She gave a knowing nod to my dropping jaw. Neither of us could believe those words had come from her mouth.

Traveling the uncharted territory of self-compassion with no particular agenda or goal, Betty was seeing herself differently, especially her maligned muffin-top. It might never be her favorite body part, she understood, but it was an important part and a family trait she shared with her mother. Not only did it insulate Betty from the cold, but her belly, like her mom's, had protected her babies in the womb.

With self-compassion practice, Betty was also feeling differently—more content, hopeful (but not jarringly optimistic), and intrinsically motivated to eat healthfully. The biggest difference and happiest surprise was twofold: she was getting where she had nearly given up going *and* she was having the time of her life.

The more I witnessed clients, like Betty and Katherine, extend kindness to themselves, the more kindness I was able to extend to myself and my clients. Compassion is positively contagious. This is very good news for an eating issues therapist like me. Patience is truly a virtue in my line of work. Before discovering the power of self-compassion, I felt more impatient than I like to admit. To be perfectly honest, it can be trying, day in and day out, listening to the same old complaints and serving up the same old supportive comments: "No, nothing, not even Valium, is quite as soothing as eating is for you now," I have been known to say. "Yes, I understand, it *does seem* hard to believe you ate the whole thing."

Therapists don masks of neutrality, but impatience can be hard to hide, especially when mixed with frustration and judgment. My mask had been slipping, but at least I wasn't as harsh as a doctor at one of the premier weight-loss institutes. She had scolded one of my clients for consuming one too many pieces of fruit! "Stop eating so much!" she told her. Clearly, comparing myself to this doctor was unwholesome, and it didn't really help.

Self-compassion moved me to try something different in my practice. Rather than ignore or avoid my own impatience, I started practicing loving-kindness and got in touch with an old friend: my impatient dieter. The next time I overate (yes, the food shrink overeats occasionally), I didn't run from her. I welcomed her back. I listened to her feelings, the ones I had tried to bury long ago, the same ones my clients try to stuff with food. I sat with my least favorite selves: self-consciousness and self-contempt. I felt the urge to escape, but I stayed put, even when dark chocolate beckoned from the cupboard.

"What you're telling me is really helpful," I told my inner dieter. "I'd forgotten how bad it feels to sit with desperation and hopelessness. I'm so sorry I ignored you for so long." She listened. "Everyone makes mistakes sometimes," I reassured us both. "We'll be OK."

Soon after our heart-to-heart, I felt better, measurably better. On my kitchen stool, I readily got back to making healthier choices. In my office easy-chair, I sat more comfortably with clients' discomfort. Realizing that their discomfort is my discomfort, that we are more alike than I had cared to admit, I was able to listen to their complaints with more curiosity and patience. Most striking, I felt new hope for the journey: my clients' and my own. It suddenly seemed so clear and simple and true: when clients get the care and understanding they need—from others, and more importantly, from themselves—they find their way. When I get the care and understanding we all need, I get where I'm going.

I could wax on about the circuitous nature of journeys, the value of missteps and mistakes. I could make the case that everyone goes through painful moments of body hatred, even celebrities and celebrated feminists. I could quote Kirstie Alley: "I've hated myself. I've loathed myself. If I had a whip, I'd whip myself!" I could quote Gloria Steinem: "In my own mind, I am still a fat brunette from Toledo, and I always will be." But you have waited long enough. It's your turn now. You can practice the very same meditations and visualizations that helped transform Betty, Katherine, and other clients, and see for yourself what a difference self-compassion makes. In chapter 2, it's all there for the taking, including my Compassionate-Eating Quiz. Onward!

LOVING-KINDNESS SUGGESTIONS FOR CULTIVATING COMPASSION

When I write of hunger, I am really writing about love and the hunger for it, and warmth and the love of it and it is all one.

M. F. K. FISHER

New clients try to convince me that punishing discipline is the only road to permanent weight loss. They're all for self-compassion after they reach their desired weight, but not one pound sooner. Understanding that they wouldn't be sitting on my couch if self-punishment worked, I invite them to do the opposite, to try a little tenderness. That way, they can clearly see what a difference compassion makes. In this chapter, I invite you to do the same, the very same practices that have helped my clients cultivate self-compassion and lose weight naturally, without dieting or squeezing themselves into a one-size-fits-all slimming strategy.

When I talk about the difference compassion makes, I am talking about the measurable difference—to mood, outlook, eating, and yes, weight loss—that comes with practice over time. Am I saying you can actually measure self-compassion? Absolutely. There are more and less scientific measures. I refer clients interested in a scientifically accurate measure to self-compassion.org, where they can take psychologist Kristin Neff's test "How Self-Compassionate Are You?"[1] There they will find a home version of the assessment tool that Neff and other psychology researchers use in the laboratory. Like before-and-after photos, comparing this and next month's scores can be illuminating, motivating, life-changing. Other clients are just as happy to take my less scientific quiz, which I have included in this book. Jean's Compassionate-Eating Quiz assesses the same personality traits as Neff's, but it's shorter and thus more convenient. Plus, it's tailored to waist watchers. While Neff's test assesses self-compassion across the board, my quiz measures attitudes toward food, hunger, body image, and other weight-related concerns. You don't need a PhD to ace my test; the more compassionate answers are pretty much no-brainers. So resist the impulse to outwit the quiz maker, and respond as honestly as you can. That way, you will get the clearest picture of exactly how self-compassionate you are.

QUIZ 1
Jean's Compassionate-Eating Quiz

This quiz measures your current state of self-compassion by helping you assess your mental, emotional, and physical reaction to diet, weight, and body image. When you can find a quiet moment away from distractions, take a pen or pencil and sit down to reflect on how compassionate you are toward yourself. After taking the quiz, cultivate self-compassion by doing the six practices that follow at least once, if not twice, and retake the quiz. Compare the two scores and see the measurable difference that self-compassion makes over the course of just a few weeks.

Check eight statements that come closest to reflecting your general experience.

_____   1. When I eat something "bad," like a donut, I can't stop thinking about how I've blown it.

_____ 2. After an indulgent weekend, I trust myself to rein in my eating.

✓ 3. I often feel alone with my eating issues, but I know I'm not.

✓ 4. When I eat junk food, I try not to beat myself up too much.

_____ 5. I may feel uncomfortable if I'm bloated or a few pounds heavier, but it doesn't stop me from enjoying social activities.

_____ 6. I might never love my body, but I know I'd like it better ten pounds lighter.

_____ 7. No one struggles with eating like I do.

✓ 8. I don't trust myself to eat when I'm hungry and stop when I'm full, but I'd like to learn.

_____ 9. I can get down on myself when I'm bloated or a few pounds heavier, but I'll still go out in baggy clothes.

_____ 10. Paying attention to my hunger makes me want to eat, so I try to ignore it.

_____ 11. I'm always interested in what my body has to say about hunger and fullness.

✓ 12. If I lose one to two pounds per week, I'll never reach my goal weight.

_____ 13. I'd like to jumpstart my weight loss with a crash diet and then eat healthfully.

✓ 14. I didn't stick to my eating plan the whole weekend; all my weight-loss efforts are for nothing.

_____ 15. When I eat something less than healthful, I try to savor it all the same.

✓ 16. I really indulged myself over the weekend; I'm afraid to step on the scale.

✓ 17. When I feel bloated or especially fat, I won't leave the house.

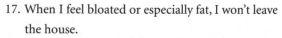

_____ 18. After overeating, I feel like punishing myself, but I
            know restricting and purging only make me feel worse.
_____ 19. Overeating is a signal to care for myself more, not less.
_____ 20. After I overeat, self-punishment (restricting food intake
            and/or purging, vomiting, or overexercising) is the only
            thing that makes me feel better.
_____ 21. My weight takes care of itself when I feed myself
            delicious, nutritious food.
___✓___ 22. When I'm overweight, I feel gross; I hate my body.
_____ 23. Everybody overeats and feels stuffed on occasion.
_____ 24. I love and respect my body.

Scoring Sheet

Give yourself 1 point per statement for checking any of the following:
1, 7, 10, 12, 14, 17, 20, 22.
Subtotal: ___4___

Give yourself 2 points per statement for checking any of the following: 3, 4, 6, 8, 9, 13, 16, 18.
Subtotal: ___8___

Give yourself 3 points per statement for checking any of the following: 2, 5, 11,15, 19, 21, 23, 24.
Subtotal: ___0___

Total Score: _12_   Date: _11_ / _27_ / _11_

Your Score and What to Make of It

When it comes to self-compassion, 0–8 means you're running on fumes;
9–16, your tank is half full; 17–24, you've got way more self-compassion
than the average American dieter. Take the test again after you've had a

chance to cultivate self-compassion, which you will learn how to do in the rest of this chapter. If your initial test score was low, you can expect the most dramatic results. You are sure to see a quantifiable leap in your score, as well as harder-to-quantify improvements, like a brighter outlook, a more upbeat mood, and a greater sense of equanimity. Even if you're already pretty kind to yourself, know that even a slight increase in self-compassion can brighten your worldview, give you more emotional balance, help you get a handle on your eating, and facilitate sustainable weight loss. (That is, if you are trying to lose weight.)

LOVING-KINDNESS SUGGESTIONS

There are many ways to cultivate self-compassion, and surely there is no one right way. In this section, you will discover a variety of traditional meditations, guided visualizations, and writing exercises that will help you generate love and acceptance of yourself. If you've opened directly to this chapter, I applaud you for following your curiosity—and I encourage you to refer back to the introduction and how to use this book when questions arise. Even if you started reading on page 1, you could probably use a recap of how to prepare yourself for practice in general. Plus, here are specific tips for the six self-compassion practices:

Ready: Find time for regular practice, ideally fifteen to twenty minutes. Most of the practices meet that minimum daily requirement, but if twenty minutes feels impossible, do several short sessions over the course of the day. You can shorten every practice, even the writing exercise, by doing a part of it, or by quickly but mindfully running through the entirety of the exercise. Of course, you can also lengthen a practice session. More is definitely better; you can't overdose on compassion. And whatever time of day you practice, you can't go wrong. While it helps to schedule practice sessions, the best time to practice is whenever you're moved to cultivate a compassionate mind-set.

Set: Find a practice-friendly space that's safe, solitary, and serene—anywhere you can comfortably sit or lie back and breathe easy. If you can get comfortable on a meditation cushion, by all means do so. But you can also relax in an armchair, on a couch, or a mat. Feel free to enhance the scene's serenity by lighting candles or incense, or wrapping yourself in a shawl or afghan.

Practice: There are dozens of ways to cultivate loving-kindness. To help you find your favorite ways, I have provided a real assortment, including my all-time favorite, metta. Some practices are short and sweet, others take more time and effort. If the first ones seem easier than the last few, they are, because I have ordered them by level of challenge. Try all six of the practices at least once, mentally noting those you find most beneficial.

The first time through a practice, read the introduction, and stick closely to the script. Once you've got the gist of the shorter practices, you can set aside the scripts and mentally guide yourself with closed eyes if you like. For the longer practices, you will need to meditate on the words with open eyes, or enlist an actual or virtual guide—a friend to read you a script, or a device that can play your reading voice. If you prefer, you can let *The Self-Compassion Diet* audio be your guide.

Once you're familiar with the various practices, don't hesitate to adjust the fit. Like a pair of jeans, you can squeeze yourself into an uncomfortable style or you can opt for a more relaxed fit. For example, if you prefer writing to visualizing, turn the guided visualizations into journal entries. If you can't sit still, try standing or walking if it makes sense. Whatever your practice style, when distractions inevitably interrupt your focus and your breathing rhythm, remember to acknowledge the distraction, refocus on the rhythmic rise and fall of your belly or another vital aspect of your breathing, and pick up where you left off. When you've finished practicing, keep breathing, and take a moment to reflect on your experience and reorient yourself to your surroundings.

PRACTICE 1
Metta: Loving-Kindness Meditation

From Buddha's lips to modern-day bestselling books, metta or lov-ing-kindness meditation has literally traveled around the world and through time. This ancient practice continues to flourish because of enthusiastic practitioners like meditation instructor Sharon Salzberg, one of the first to bring this Eastern tradition to the Western reading public with her '90s bestseller, *Lovingkindness: The Revolutionary Art of Happiness.* To reap the benefits, you don't need to become a medita-tion scholar, but you could do with a mini-history lesson.

Buddha first prescribed metta as an antidote to fear. As the story goes, a gang of tree spirits spooked some monks who were trying to meditate in the forest. Rather than suggest a more peaceable spot, the compassionate leader insisted the monks return to the forest armed only with metta. This was before reality TV, so there was no big cash prize, but a more valuable, less quantifiable payoff: courage. Fast-forward to the finale: not only did metta quell the monks' fears, it inspired the tree spirits to adopt a more altruistic livelihood—pro-tecting and serving the monks. That's right, the whole forest profited from that initial investment in loving-kindness. The take-home lesson is clear, and becomes clearer with regular practice. Loving-kindness is good for what ails you. As soon as you feel better, you'll want to pay it forward to family, friends, even complete strangers.

Meditation often focuses the attention on the breath, but metta focuses on phrases. Begin by adopting a caring attitude as if you were singing a lullaby to a distressed child. Then silently repeat the follow-ing phrases:

May I be safe
May I be happy
May I be healthy
May I live with ease

Next, imagine sending loving-kindness to a loved one:

> *May you be safe*
> *May you be happy*
> *May you be healthy*
> *May you live with ease*

Finally, envision a larger group—all your loved ones, all women who struggle with eating issues, the human race—and repeat:

> *May we be safe*
> *May we be happy*
> *May we be healthy*
> *May we live with ease*

The above phrases are traditional, but feel free to shorten them to mantras or prayerful words: "safe," "happy," "healthy," "ease." Or a single mantra. If, given your life circumstances, "healthy" and "happy" seem like a stretch, focus on "safety" or "ease." If the phrases don't work as written, rewrite them. Add a word or two: May I [learn to] be healthy. May I [learn to] be happy, and so forth. Distill the message into fewer lines. Or consider using three especially lovely phrases by Cambridge Insight Meditation Center metta instructor Narayan Liebenson Grady:[2]

> *May I have peace of mind*
> *May I have openness of heart*
> *May I be fully at ease*

If you prefer writing your own phrases, take all the poetic license you like. The idea is to compose short, personally meaningful statements that capture the universal wish for happiness and freedom from suffering. An easy way to start writing, especially if you're in the habit of telling yourself mean, nasty things, is to write the opposite of one of the meaner, nastier things you tell yourself. For example, the antithesis to reminding yourself that your weight is unacceptable could be: *May I learn to accept myself as I am, at least in this moment.*

If you can't imagine sending yourself a single self-compassionate word, take a play from Chris Germer's playbook, *The Mindful Path to Self-Compassion.*[3] Sneak up on yourself with kindness! Start by sending loving-kindness to a pet, a child, someone undeniably lovable, and insert yourself into the meditation as soon as you can:

> *May Fido walk in peace*
> *May all beings walk in peace*
> *Me, too*

Or:

> *May my daughter set aside shame and accept her body*
> *May my daughter and I set aside shame and accept our bodies*
> *May all women set aside shame and accept their bodies*

Metta's focus may be words, but expanding your focus to include imagery, feelings, and sensations enriches the experience. Notice what happens when you zoom in on the true meaning of the words, the details of the visualization, the sensation of your heartbeat, the emotions that arise. You might expect loving-kindness meditation to inspire warm, fuzzy feelings. Sometimes it does. Other times, well, don't be surprised if you bump into difficult feelings (boredom, sadness, impatience), uncomfortable sensations (pain, itchiness, antsy-ness), or sad memories.

NO STUPID QUESTIONS

Q Isn't it selfish to cultivate self-compassion?

A Just the opposite! Self-compassion practices are exercises in generosity. Think of self-compassion like oxygen in an airplane emergency: when you help yourself first, you're better able to take care of those in need.

No need to run from the experience if—I should say *when*—you meet discomfort. You've got choices. If the experience feels tolerable, stay with it. Your discomfort will likely change, if not pass. If you get lost in a swamp of thought or feeling, however, seek refuge in the breath or the "I" phrases: *May I be safe . . .* If your swamp becomes physically uncomfortable, treat yourself kindly. Adjust your position or continue the practice standing or walking. Walking metta is a refreshing change of pace, especially when practiced outdoors. Alternate between sending loving-kindness to yourself and whoever crosses your path—dogs, bicyclists, the homeless.

It's also your call how long you devote to the objects of your compassion. If you've only got five minutes, send metta to a dying parent, a divorcing friend, a laid-off colleague—the person who needs it most. If that person is you, set aside fears of selfishness and dedicate the practice to you. The formal practice calls for sending metta to a longer list of recipients—a "benefactor," a mentor, or anyone who inspires deep gratitude; a "neutral person," someone you see, but don't really know, such as the Chihuahua owner at the dog park or a colleague in a distant cubicle; and an "enemy," a difficult person who invites conflict, inspires distress, or knows how to push your buttons.

If at any point you want to learn more about metta or any of the practices, chapter 9 will teach you how. Right now, repeat after me: *May I be safe . . .*

PRACTICE 2

Compassionate Advisor: A Guided Visualization

The Compassionate Advisor Visualization is a tried-and-true technique for easing all manner of human suffering. That this visualization is prescribed in such a wide variety of settings—meditation centers, religious sanctuaries, mental-health clinics, hypnotherapy offices, psychiatric hospitals, cancer wards—is a testament to the power of the practice. Many well-known health practitioners have introduced the Compassionate Advisor to their patients—such as Martin Rossman, the California physician who made his name helping cancer survivors, among others, ease their physical and emotional pain with a little help from this practice; and Paul Gilbert, the British research psychologist who developed Compassionate Mind Training, an established treatment for eating disorders. According to preliminary findings, bulimics who practice this and other compassion-enhancing techniques boost their recovery rate from 50 to 70 percent.[4]

Like loving-kindness meditation, the content of this visualization may vary from session to session, but the underlying assumption remains the same—a wise, compassionate advisor or guide lives within us all.[5] In a world that has outsourced wisdom to experts with advanced degrees and fancy initials, it's easy to disregard your own inner wisdom. This practice is an opportunity to consult the expert who knows you best: you.

Take a moment to find a comfortable position and a natural breathing rhythm. Allow your breath to naturally deepen as you inhale, and lengthen as you exhale. When you're ready, call to mind a wise, compassionate advisor, the embodiment of kindness and gentleness. It could be a character direct from central casting (a wizard, a mountain-dwelling monk), or a beloved religious figure (Buddha, Jesus). It could be an embodiment of compassion from the past (Mother Teresa, Gandhi) or present (the Dalai Lama), or a benevolent fictional character (Yoda, Jiminy Cricket), or a wise bestselling author (Geneen Roth, Maya Angelou). It could also be someone "close to home": a caring relative or a loving pet. Your imagination is limitless; your guide can take any form (animal, tree, mountain, ocean) or no form (a healing light or energy).

As the mind focuses on one image or idea, invite the senses to bring your advisor to life. If seeing is a strong sense for you, notice what your guide looks like. Notice as many visual details as you can. If your advisor appears as a living being, note gender, age, clothing, posture, facial expression . . . whatever you can. If your advisor takes the form of an inanimate object, notice its size, shape, color, texture, and so on. If you tend to absorb information through your feelings, pay attention to how it feels to be near this compassionate being, to feel your guide's love, strength, and patience. If hearing is your dominant sense, focus on the sound of your advisor's voice—caring, soothing, reassuring. Whether you use one or more senses, let yourself absorb your advisor's essential qualities. Allow yourself to soak up what's so hard to come by in everyday life: unconditional acceptance. There's nothing quite like the ease that comes with unconditional acceptance.

Your all-knowing advisor is aware of your concerns, and it's always worthwhile to give your concerns the care and attention they deserve. Take the time to focus on what concerns you the most, then ask for what you need: support, guidance, advice. Or maybe advice is the last thing you need. Maybe what you most need right now is relief from suffering, confusion, or despair. Give your guide time and space to deliver on your request by continuing to breathe and focus. Help might arrive immediately or sometime later. Wisdom takes its own sweet time. And it can take different forms—a sudden "aha," a revealing image, an accepting feeling, a quiet inner voice of knowing, a new perspective. However help manifests, let yourself receive it.

If you don't get everything you need, ask for more, receive more. Don't hesitate to ask for more clarity, answers, or support—everything you need. If what you receive leaves you wanting more, ask for another consultation. The advisor is always in. There will be many chances to get perspective, guidance, and support. It's time to say thank you, and good-bye for now. To take a deep breath and make your way back to this moment. Wiser and calmer. Kinder and gentler. Here and now.

Put Self-Compassion on Trial

Is your inner jury still out on the case of self-compassion for weight loss? I invite you to put self-compassion on trial, enlisting yourself as expert witness. The next time you polish off a pint of Chunky Monkey or make a less-than-healthful food choice, forgo self-recrimination and consider getting an imaginary opinion or two. For the first opinion, imagine a real-life harsh critic (a judgmental boss, an unfeeling acquaintance) or a storybook character (a wicked witch, a cruel stepmother) insulting you for overeating. Try as you might, it's impossible to ignore the insults about your sinful behavior and glaring flaws.

Okay, that's enough scolding. Take a deep breath and notice how hopeful you feel about getting back to making healthy dietary decisions. Then get a second opinion. Imagine your compassionate advisor from the previous practice or another kind soul—a therapist, favorite relative, historic or fictional character—helping you better understand and cope. Have an imaginary discussion with this loving being, or just listen to your advisor's caring words. Take as much time as you need to view yourself from this caring viewpoint, weigh the evidence, and reach a verdict.

Cruelty or compassion: which promises to free you from the prison of overeating? What say ye?

Compassionate Note to Self: A Writing Exercise

For people who find writing therapeutic, this journaling practice is a great way to cultivate self-compassion and relaxation.[6] A compassionate letter a day just might keep the body hatred away. That's right, committing your deepest concerns to paper is scientifically proven to bolster positive emotional mind-sets and weaken negative mental states.

To be clear, the practice of composing a compassionate note to self is not to avoid or replace therapy or other supports you may or may not have. Rather, writing yourself a love letter is another way of tending to your emotional wounds with care and attention.

To do this exercise, you'll need a comfortable space, pen and paper, and a clear surface you can call your own for fifteen to twenty minutes of uninterrupted writing. (You can do this practice typing on a computer keyboard, but the primal act of writing by hand is somehow more powerful and empowering.)

Before you put pen to paper, first deepen your breathing, set aside concerns about grammar and spelling, and flip through your mental Rolodex of distressing situations, unsettling interactions, and other emotion-packed events in your recent history. Choose one event or interaction that has caused you angst. As you recall the who, what, when, where, and why of the scenario, let yourself remember all you can about what you were thinking, doing, and feeling.

Now imagine a loving being—a living, breathing loved one, a caring character who lives in your imagination, or your compassionate advisor from the last practice, anyone who knows what you most need to hear. As words of comfort and concern come to mind, begin writing yourself a letter from this imaginary pen pal. Let the words flow from pen to paper, conveying whatever you need: support, perspective, forgiveness, advice, a reminder of something you already know. Maybe this friend has something to share about perfection—that you don't have to be perfect, that your imperfections make you more, not less, lovable.

If laughter is your best medicine, don't be afraid to use humor: "You made a mistake? You're human! Join the club!" If you like truisms, and they not only ring true but truly soothe, use them, too: "Time heals all wounds"; "This too will pass"; "One day at a time." If careful analysis is more your style, write about demographics, genetics, family, culture, the media—all the sociological factors that have contributed to your concern. "You're predisposed to eating issues," you might write. "You hail from a long line of overeaters. You are surely not alone." But if you prefer psychological explanations, your letter writing might focus on strengths and weaknesses, and the challenge of replacing destructive habits with more constructive ones.

When you've conveyed all you need to convey, sign the note if you like, and set aside your pen and paper. Give yourself the necessary time and space to breathe, to reflect, and to feel.

Writing about personal concerns offers reliable relief, but not instantly. Don't be surprised if this writing exercise stirs you up before it calms you down. If you like, read your letter aloud to yourself or someone you trust. Conversely, if you're moved to tear it up and throw it away, do so. What's most therapeutic is the act of writing, not reading. Over and over, translating your deepest concerns into the written word will help you cultivate compassion.

PRACTICE 4
Compassionate Glasses: A Guided Visualization

Dieters unhappy with the fit of their jeans have been known to ask their near and dear ones: "Do I look fat?" It matters little what the scale says. In this desperate state, the person asking the no-win question fears that they have suddenly ballooned. Because harsh judgment distorts body image more cruelly than a fun-house mirror, it's difficult for the dieter to get an accurate assessment in the mirror. So they ask: "Do I look fat?"

The correct answer is something warm and fuzzy, not the cold, hard truth. Something like: "You don't have a good sense of your actual size or any idea how beautiful you are." Too many significant others make the mistake of answering the question literally, and paying for it dearly. They say, "Your butt has never been your best feature, and now that you mention it, it has gotten bigger." Some have wised up and learned to withhold their opinion, or turn their response into a loving and empowering statement. Often, silence proves less than helpful because it fails to answer the real, unarticulated question: "Can you spare some compassion?"

I developed this visualization to help clients give themselves the compassion they desperately need in order to soften their

self-judgment and interrupt the vicious cycle that too often cul-
minates in front of the refrigerator, the pantry, the all-you-can-eat
buffet.[7] For this practice, you will need two pairs of imaginary
glasses—one with distorted lenses, and one more compassionate
pair. The distorted perspective is all too familiar and clearly painful,
but it makes the contrasting view even more powerful. Most clients
find both perspectives instructive. If the first proves to be too much,
go directly to the second, more compassionate one. It's healing in
and of itself.

Once you have settled into a relaxed pose and a quiet breathing
rhythm, imagine trying on glasses with distorted lenses—a pair that
allows you to see yourself in the worst possible light. The frames
aren't particularly stylish, the view may not be all that clear, but take
an imaginary look at yourself in an old, tarnished, full-length mirror. Whether you see yourself clothed or naked, focus on your least
favorite body parts. If you have recently gained weight, notice where
you have gained it. Linger on the bulges, the sags, the cellulite, all
the visual imperfections. Expand your focus to include self-critical
thoughts: "If I'd stuck to my diet, I'd be thinner and happier. I've
really blown it!" Let yourself ruminate on all that's wrong: "I hate my
body. It's gross. I'll never lose weight. It's hopeless!" Invite self-pity:
"Other people lose weight; why can't I? There must be something
wrong with me." While it may be tempting to switch glasses, stick
with this pair until you feel more than a little agitated, but less than
completely miserable.

Now try on the other glasses, the pair with the compassionate lenses.
Exhaling discomfort, inhaling calm, take another look at yourself, this
time in a crystal-clear, full-length mirror. Take a good look at your
whole body in the mirror's beautiful golden light. You're glowing with
natural energy. As you drink in your reflection, allow compassion to
wash over you, refreshing and relaxing you at the same time. Whether

you're clothed or naked, notice what a difference compassion makes. It's easier, isn't it, to appreciate your health and vitality with loving eyes? It's hard to ignore the marvelous design of the human body, your body. Your inner beauty. Your head and heart. Your innate ability to think, to feel, to love. It's only natural to stand tall, with dignity and confidence.

It is not that you must see total perfection when you look at your body and being with compassionate eyes. You can see beauty in your imperfections. Or at the very least, you can view your body with more acceptance, less criticism. You can see your least favorite body parts with the pride and gratitude of a new mother. You are grateful for all that's right: toes and fingers, eyes and ears, lips that can smile, a being that can experience laughter and enjoy all that life has to offer.

In this glorious light, your body is undeniably a temple, worthy of care and protection, deserving of delicious, nutritious food. Some body fat is necessary: it keeps you warm and comfortable. It sustains you in sickness and in health. Your compassionate lenses are without distortion. You can see that as clearly as you can see your true shape. You can see overeating for the sign that it is: the need to pay attention. To pay attention to how you feel, what you need, if you want support. Everyone overeats sometimes; it's normal. If you notice you've been overeating too often, it's clear in this light that something's asking for your attention. Whatever's asking for your attention, it's definitely worth attending to.

Of course, you can always eat better, exercise more regularly. That's part of taking good care of yourself. But it's not the whole picture. You can see the big picture with your compassionate

THINK SELF-KIND THOUGHTS

Your Inner Critic:
I'll never lose weight. I'm
_____ *(fill in a personal put-down)*.

Your Compassionate Response:
_____
_____
_____
_____

glasses. You've got perspective. What stands out is how pleasing it is to view yourself through kinder, gentler eyes; to actually *embody* a greater sense of calm, well-being, and patience. There is a wonderful ease that comes with greater self-acceptance and a more balanced viewpoint.

Because you enjoy this viewpoint, you might like to prescribe yourself an imaginary pair of contact lenses. Lenses that allow you to take this warmer, more benevolent view of yourself with you wherever you go, that allow you to take this renewed sense of positive self-regard with you.

PRACTICE 5
Head-to-Toe Appreciation: A Guided Visualization

This consciousness-raising practice might have come of age during the Women's Movement, but it survives because it transforms the way we view our bodies, ourselves.[8] The "sixties' version" called for facing the naked truth in a full-length mirror by surveying your bare body as if it were a work of art—from head to toe, with eyes wide open, appreciating its sculptural dimensions, shape, texture, and color. *If* you were willing to stare down the self-loathing and other negative feelings that American women harbor toward the female body, the original practice could be empowering. But that was and still is a big *if.*

Pained by their unadulterated reflection, some dieters are unwilling to try the newer, gentler variations of this practice—even when fully clothed. For some, the very idea of taking a good, hard look in the looking glass is unimaginable. With Pema Chödrön's words of wisdom in mind—"Just start where you are"—I developed a kinder, gentler version of this classic visualization, to be done with eyes comfortably closed. There's no dress code. Do it wearing whatever, including if you like the compassionate contacts from the last practice.

When you've settled into a comfortable position and a quiet breathing rhythm, imagine your body clothed or naked—not an idealized image of your body as it once was or will be again, but your present shape. Without judgment, drink in your reflection as objectively as you can. If and when self-criticism arises, refocus on the breath and a more objective viewpoint.

From head to toe, let your mind count the ways each body part serves you. Your hair shields you from the weather, keeps you warm, and come to think of it, boosts your mood on great hair days. Your skull protects your brain. Wax poetic if you like: your eyes are the windows to the world. Or stick to the facts: your neck supports your head. Your teeth play an important role in chewing, speaking, smiling. Arms make hugging possible. Your shoulders do the heavy lifting, carry a knapsack, give piggyback rides.

Take extra care with body parts that magazines promise to shape up in no time—your stomach, thighs, and behind. Unless it's sustained you in illness or protected you in an accident, it can be hard to imagine how belly fat serves you, but it does serve you. If you're a mom or expecting to be one, consider how your body makes mothering possible. Your pelvis protects babies before they're born, your breasts nourish them afterward. If you're a dad or a dad-to-be, you might consider how the magic of your body allows for your child to come into being.

When you finish recounting everything your body does to serve and protect you, step back for one last look. One final full-length view of your reflection. With fresh eyes, reflect on the sum that's far greater than the individual parts. With this heightened awareness, pause to appreciate the living, breathing miracle of the human body. Linger a little longer in mindful awareness of the breath and your renewed appreciation of your body.

Eat Like a Bird

Waist watchers talk about "guilty pleasures," but in my professional opinion, there's no such thing. If you've ever eaten something you thought you "shouldn't," you know how cruel guilt can be. How it eventually robs pleasure from your eating experience. How so-called transgressions punish you for hours, days, maybe weeks after you've swallowed the last tasty morsel. How guilt's trash-talking sidekick, self-loathing, compels you to seek refuge in yet another guilty pleasure.

If you'd like to break this vicious, hopeless cycle, eat like a bird. Let me explain: as they flit around bird feeders, sparrows, robins, and their feathered neighbors make every meal a songfest. Come dinnertime, they peck and chirp, chirp and peck. Even when it's standing room only at the bird feeder, they're savoring and singing in unison. What they're not squawking about is their weight. The same can be said of ducks in duckweed, seagulls on clam flats. Our fine feathered friends make a persuasive case: food is something to sing about.

Another great way to cast guilt to the wind is listening to musicians from the Louisiana bayou, who wax melodic about "jambalaya, crawfish pie, filé gumbo." Or reading vintage essays by the late food writer Laurie Colwin: "One of the delights of life is eating with friends, second to that is talking about eating. And, for an unsurpassed double whammy, there is talking about eating while you are eating with friends."

PRACTICE 6
Tonglen: Give-and-Take Meditation

Just as metta has the potential to turn self-hatred into self-love, *tonglen* transforms human suffering into altruism.[9] Often considered a more advanced practice than metta, tonglen (also known as give-and-take meditation) invites you to override your natural instincts and do something that, at least initially, feels completely unnatural—*take* in your least favorite feelings and *give* away your most. You read right: breathe in your own suffering, and breathe out emotional relief to others who suffer similarly. If you were to feel bored, lonely, or sad during this formal practice, you'd drink in boredom, loneliness, or sadness, and pour out interest, companionship, or happiness. If you were practicing informally in your office cubicle, you'd sit with your midafternoon exhaustion and send vitality to colleagues circling the Coke machine. A better name for this exercise might be take-and-give practice, because you're really *taking in* pain, *giving back* care.

This ancient Tibetan meditation may sound like the definition of masochism, but psychotherapists prescribe tonglen to clients who struggle with anxiety and other troubling symptoms. Because when you stop running away and start turning toward a feared feeling, you get used to it. Or, in therapy-speak, you "habituate" to it. In the moment, you might think you would prefer fleeting pleasure to enduring distress. You might believe you would rather hide your head in a bag of Doritos than face your self-consciousness in a three-way mirror. But you really don't. Why? Because you and I both know that stuffing feelings backfires big-time! Over time, stuffed feelings get more persistent and fierce, fierce enough to undermine the best-laid weight-loss plans.

More effectively than other practices, tonglen tames fierce emotions, including those that unleash emotional eating. But not overnight. Tonglen takes practice and care. Begin practicing with mild distress, and over time work up to increasingly intense feelings. The script below will show you how to start slowly, surely, symbolically.

As soon as you settle into a comfortable position, focus on the rhythm of your breathing. Take a full, deep inhalation with intention, and then hold your breath in silence for four seconds. Slowly exhale with a long out-breath to the count of eight seconds. As you inhale, slowly inflate your abdomen like a balloon. As you exhale, quietly deflate that balloon. Sit in silence, quietly breathing, until you find a steady rhythm with your breath.

When you're ready, imagine inhaling darkness, exhaling light. Darkness is suffering—black and heavy. Light is healing—white and airy. As you inhale, take in hot, heavy blackness. As you exhale, send out light, cool whiteness. If the pace feels rushed, slow it down. Focus on darkness for several breath cycles before you switch to light.

Once you've got the rhythm and the spirit of the practice, shift your attention from breathing to feeling. If you're new to tonglen, notice or invite in a feeling that's a little uncomfortable, but not overwhelming. If mild emotional discomfort isn't readily available, bring to mind a recent irritation—a choice comment, a thoughtless e-mail, a traffic jam. Drink in the mix of uncomfortable feelings; pour a better brew for your irritated sisters around the world. You might inhale annoyance, exhale calm. Or breathe in pettiness, breathe out generosity.

If at any point you feel reluctant to continue this practice, or eager to move on to other things, know that you are not alone. Breathe in reluctance; breathe out willingness. Keep taking in reluctance and giving back willingness, or staying with whatever pair of feelings you're giving and taking. Stay with the practice for a set length of time or until the intensity of the uncomfortable feeling noticeably decreases—until you are, in fact, breathing easier.

You have started working with mild annoyance, but the ultimate goal of tonglen is taking on the deepest suffering of all beings. Not to worry: achieving a healthy, sustainable weight doesn't require taking on the world's woes. Your own problems will do just fine.

Now that you have learned six different ways to cultivate self-compassion, six great alternatives to punitive self-discipline, rather than rushing off to the next chapter, consider staying put. Maybe revisiting some, if not all, of the above practices. Actively appreciating and accepting yourself for a little while longer, until you actually feel a little more appreciative and accepting. When you do, don't forget to retake the Compassionate-Eating Quiz to confirm your measurable progress. Validate your self-caring efforts.

PART II

Hypnosis

The Power of Positive Suggestion

THE ENCHANTING
HYPNOTHERAPIST

Once you realize that willpower is just a matter
of learning how to control your attention and
thoughts, you can really begin to increase it.

WALTER MISCHEL

Hypnosis, the first slimming route I explored as a young psychotherapist, is the most requested weight-loss method in my private practice. And yet, when I tell people that I make much of my living hypnotizing clients slim, they still ask: "Does it work?" My answer usually brightens their eyes with something between excitement and incredulity. Most people, including my colleagues at Harvard Medical School, don't realize that adding trance to your weight-loss efforts can help you lose more weight and keep it off longer—long enough to establish healthy eating habits.

Hypnosis predates carb and calorie counting by a few centuries—dating back to when Franz Mesmer, the forefather of modern-day hypnosis, was curing what ailed the French elite in the late 1700s. But this age-old attention-focusing technique has yet to be embraced wholeheartedly as an effective weight-loss strategy.

Until recently, there has been scant scientific evidence to support the legitimate claims of respected hypnotherapists, and a glut of pie-in-the-sky promises from their problem cousins, stage hypnotists, hasn't helped. (No, hypnotists don't have the power to make you cluck like a chicken. Truth be told, hypnotic subjects who do goofy things on stage volunteer knowing full well what's expected: entertainment.) Even after a persuasive re-analysis of the best hypnotic studies showed that psychotherapy clients who learned self-hypnosis lost twice as much weight as those who didn't, hypnotherapy has remained a weight-loss secret. Unless hypnosis has happily propelled you or someone you know to buy a new, smaller wardrobe, it may be hard to believe that this mind-over-body approach could help you get a handle on your eating. Seeing is definitely believing!

HYPNOSIS 101

There may be as many answers to the question of "What is hypnosis?" as there are for the eternal head-scratcher "What is love?" Some answers are better than others, and one pretty good one is the official definition from the American Society of Clinical Hypnosis, the largest professional organization for health-care providers using clinical hypnosis: "Hypnosis is a state of inner absorption, concentration, and focused attention. It is like using a magnifying glass to focus the rays of the sun and make them more powerful. Similarly, when our minds are concentrated and focused, we are able to use our minds more powerfully. Because hypnosis allows people to use more of their potential, learning self-hypnosis is the ultimate act of self-control." [1]

To be perfectly honest, hypnosis is rather mysterious. Psychologists have dedicated careers to pinpointing what happens during hypnosis—to the brain, body, sense of self—but there is no single, uncontestable truth about what it is and why it's so powerful. Many of my esteemed colleagues, however, would say that the power of hypnosis lies within the subject. The hypnotist may suggest that a client focus her attention and cultivate relaxation in order to travel inward and harness the power of the unconscious, but the subject controls the trance's depth and direction. All hypnosis is essentially self-hypnosis.

Hypnotherapists, the psychotherapists who practice hypnosis, can't agree on much else, but most can and do agree on one thing: hypnosis works. It works best when performed by licensed health-care providers, including clinicial psychologists, medical doctors, and social workers who have gotten at least a year of postgraduate training in the theory and practice of hypnosis. It's a lot less effective when practiced by taxi drivers, hairdressers, and other unlicensed practitioners who have taken a crash course in stage hypnosis. Clients would wholeheartedly agree on hypnotherapy's effectiveness, but have their own ideas about how it works. One client who lost 35 pounds came to understand hypnosis to be all about the second syllable: hyp-*no*-sis. When this forty-year-old realtor makes time for trance, he finds it easy to say *no* to a third slice of pizza, *no* to another round of drinks, and *no* to empty calories.

What's clear as new contact lenses is what hypnosis is not. It's not magic. It's not a cure-all. The word "hypnosis" comes from the Greek word for sleep (*hypnos*), but besides closed eyes and the characteristic relaxed position, the hypnotic experience is far from sleep and the furthest thing from the coma-like state portrayed in movies. The immobilizing spell that comes over countless fictional characters is another bad stereotype that perpetuates popular misconceptions. Unlike Emerald City-bound Dorothy, who gets very sleeeeeeeppy in that psychedelic poppy field, or Snow White, who falls into a deep stupor after one apple bite, hypnotic subjects are not only alert during trance, they can talk, walk, even eat. After they reawaken—or more accurately, re-alert themselves—they can remember.

The words "trance" and "hypnosis" are often lumped together even by professional therapists, but it's worth unlumping them. Simply put, hypnosis is a therapeutic tool for mining inner strengths and abilities

that helped you reach goals in the past. Another favorite analogy: hypnosis is a vehicle for speeding around familiar obstacles and past pitfalls
to your desired destination—without a crash collision. Like a pizza
delivery van, the vehicle of hypnosis helps me quickly deliver the most
effective and palatable treatment for the full range of eating problems.
Like pizza toppings, clients order from a menu of slimming strategies.
Then they relax, and I serve their order with personal attention and care.

If hypnosis is the pizza van, trance is the pizza-eating experience—a sensual feast, an all-consuming delight that requires no
formalities, but can be enjoyed day or night, in more and less formal
settings. In other words, trance can happen under different circumstances in many different places, both informally and formally. In a
hypnotherapist's office where you consciously alter your mental focus
and emotional state, that's formal trance. In daydreams and fantasies
when you subconsciously shift your attention and feeling state, that's
informal trance. In formal trance, the hypnotherapist intentionally
focuses a client's attention, then offers tailor-made suggestions and
images to the receptive unconscious mind. With informal trance, the
shift in focus happens unassisted and unintentionally, such as when
you're driving on autopilot, getting lost in a good book or movie,
playing a sport or a musical instrument with more ease and grace
than you could deliberately. As we go about our day, we all naturally
go in and out of trance.

Some hypnotists try to capture the je ne sais quoi of this mysterious
experience in a simple phrase, like "state of mind" or "altered state of
consciousness." Others go to great lengths to accurately define trance
with a checklist of specific traits and predictable phenomena. The latter, more scientific-minded group has developed standardized scales,
like the Stanford Hypnotic Susceptibility Scale and the Harvard
Group Scale of Hypnotic Susceptibility, to measure hypnotic ability or "hypnotizability." If you were a fly on one of these researchers'

walls, you could observe any number of phenomenal changes in subjects' behavior (arms floating in mid-air, feet seemingly superglued to
the floor), physiology (blood flow starting and stopping on cue), and
feeling (subjects spontaneously smiling or giggling). Objective measures are useful in the lab, but have by no means solved the puzzle that
is trance. It remains one of life's unsolved mysteries, right up there
with the Bermuda Triangle and the land of lost socks.

When hypnosis is used as a therapeutic tool, a client's subjective
experience matters more than her objective responsiveness. Outside
the lab, standardized tests are rarely used to grade hypnotizability.
And yet, the question on the tip of most clients' tongues—"Will this
work?"—suggests they expect to be graded at least pass-fail. I try to set
them straight from the get-go. There will be no grades, I tell them, just
genuine interest in any positive reaction to trance, such as enhanced
relaxation, motivation, energy, and more. A low hypnotizable who is
highly motivated can do better in therapy than an unmotivated high
hypnotizable who expects me to do all the work. Because subjective
experience defies measurement and varies not only from person to
person but from trance to trance, I tend to wax more poetic than
scientific when I explain the phenomenon of hypnosis.

THIS THANG CALLED TRANCE

To my metaphorical mind, the transformative real-life experience that
comes closest to trance is romance. In both falling in love and falling
under trance, subjects, with the help of a mesmerizing other, completely focus on the sensory-rich experience of the present moment.
In other words, they effortlessly enter the state that's just as integral
to self-compassion: mindful awareness. Just so you know, like healthy
self-love, there's also self-hypnosis.

Both trance and romance help us finally do what's so much easier
said than done—to cast off yesterday's regrets and future worries, to

dive into the power of right now. In both magical states, distractions fade away, freeing subjects to absorb themselves in deeper feelings, keener sensations, more vivid fantasies—to revel in the exhilarating experience of being fully alive. Everything that happens feels automatic and effortless. The exciting ideas and possibilities that arise unbidden are mind-blowing in the best possible way. You don't lose touch with reality when you're infatuated or entranced, but reality is markedly different. Time seems to pass more quickly, or slowly. The world looks brighter, more welcoming, quite beautiful. Beauty is always in the eye of the beholder, but when you're entranced or infatuated, it's easier to see what you want to see, and blind yourself to the rest.

Some hypnotic subjects have real talent for altering their visual perception of themselves and their surroundings. If I were to suggest that a high hypnotizable should gaze into an imaginary mirror and see her ideal reflection, it wouldn't surprise her to find a young, bikini-clad Raquel Welch. If I were then to suggest she see her true reflection, minus the freckles, she would be able to see her own familiar face, miraculously freckle-free. This superhypnotic talent comes in handy at buffets, when waist watchers intent on skipping dessert can view the dessert table and see only fake food. Believing that they're seeing a plastic food display of cheesecakes, crème brûlée, and chocolate-dipped strawberries, they can watch their cravings disappear.

Like IQ, hypnotic ability is relatively stable throughout adulthood. It has nothing to do with personality traits (passivity, gullibility), a lot to do with the ability to get absorbed (in a good conversation, a suspense novel, a knitting project), and less to do with a hypnotist's skill or a subject's motivation. Motivation *can* make subjects slightly more suggestible. Subjects who were tricked into believing they could be hypnotized (for example, when the hypnotist suggested that the subject would see red, he flipped the switch on a hidden red bulb) demonstrated increased hypnotic responsiveness. When I say "seeing is believing," what I really mean is seeing what looks like evidence of trance can boost belief and temporarily enhance responsiveness. But, and this is an important *but*, there's nothing that can substantially improve or alter hypnotic ability in any lasting way.

Hypnotic ability may be hereditary (identical twins score more alike than their fraternal counterparts on standardized tests), but on average, children are more hypnotizable than their parents. Most adults have modest to moderate ability, but a small minority have exceptional talent. Maybe you have seen one of these extremely hypnotizable adults on TV: these are the people who have C-sections or other surgical procedures without chemical anesthesia, and in some cases walk out of the hospital soon after.[2]

A HIDDEN TALENT

You might be surprised to learn that women afraid of getting fat are a supertalented bunch. Ours is a diet-crazed nation, but hypnosis studies have shown that women with an unhealthy obsession with calorie counting and waist watching are more suggestible than average. You read right: women who are hyperfocused on diet and weight, including those with eating disorders, are more susceptible to our culture's "thin is beautiful" message.[3] (When researchers get around to replicating this study with male subjects, I suspect that fat-fearing men will also prove to have above-average hypnotic abilities.)

This hidden talent is a double-edged sword. On the one edge, higher hypnotizability may actually predispose dieters to develop eating disorders. On the other, it could make them more responsive to hypnotic treatment. Ideally, fat-fearing dieters interested in treatment would find a hypnotherapist experienced in eating issues and loving-kindness meditation. Rather than fueling fears with strict dieting suggestions, the therapist could readily address the patient's eating issues, and ease their fear by offering meditative phrases as hypnotic suggestions. Hypnosis, studies have shown, significantly reduces binging and vomiting, and reliably decreases underlying body dissatisfaction and the drive for thinness.[4]

THINK SELF-KIND THOUGHTS

Your Inner Critic:
I'm afraid of getting fat. I'm afraid if I keep eating like this, I'll _____ (fill in your worst-case scenario).

Your Compassionate Response:
_____
_____
_____
_____

The average American dieter with more modest hypnotic ability can do quite well with hypnosis—and significantly better, in fact, than they can with most other weight-loss strategies. Just ask Beth. Like many veteran dieters who settle onto my couch, this fifty-seven-year-old community organizer started her story as if reading from a script: "I've tried everything. Nothing works!" Defeated dieters like Beth live with the delusion that no matter what they do, they can't lose weight. This defeated dieter easily entered trance, but despite considerable hypnotic ability, she had difficulty picturing herself at her desired weight.

Never in her wildest dreams could she have foreseen that, months later, she would tell untold millions about her metamorphosis on national TV, and that after demonstrating trance on the *CBS Evening News*, she would explain: "The suggestions are in my head; it's kind of automatic." This happier, thinner Beth went on to say: "I look at fruits and vegetables more; they're much more appealing to me." I was delighted for Beth, and not the least bit surprised by the reporter's conclusion: "Beth lost 15 pounds and she never felt like she was on a diet." I was more bewildered by the fact that the reporter, a medical doctor, was only starting to realize that hypnosis makes dieting irrelevant. Why would any waist watcher want to feel "like she was on a diet"? Why would anyone consciously choose to count calories when the unconscious mind is more than willing to do the menu planning?

PERSONAL SLIMMING LESSON

Forbid This, Not That?

A list of forbidden foods, many dieters believe, is the answer to their dieting prayers. They desperately want an authority to tell them what to eat, what to eliminate. And the willpower to do what Eve failed to do: just say no. That diet authorities keep changing their minds about what's forbidden and what's not doesn't detract from the popularity of these lists. If Eve sought nutritional advice today, she would eliminate high-fructose corn syrup, not apples. Does forbidding yourself certain foods encourage or discourage you from eating healthfully? That is the question.

Before you consider eliminating anything from your diet, try this quick experiment. Bring to mind a yummy high-calorie indulgence. In your mind's eye, see it, taste it, savor every last bite. Now, as you have probably done countless times before, tell yourself: never again. NO MORE. Mentally forbid yourself this indulgence. Ban it from your diet and your thoughts. Seriously, don't think about it. For the next minute, set aside all thoughts of this treat. Sixty seconds, 59, 58 . . . give yourself a full minute . . . How did you do NOT thinking about your forbidden fruit? Did what you resist get more or less persistent? As radical as it might sound, consider letting *your* answer be your guide.

A WINNING COMBINATION

I didn't need a Ouija board to predict Beth's success, because hers was textbook. Week in and week out, my clients demonstrate what researchers have shown time and again. Hypnosis makes weight loss easier, more doable, especially when it's combined with cognitive-behavioral therapy (CBT), the psychotherapy that helps override undermining thoughts and behaviors. Clients who learn both therapies can lose twice as much weight without falling into the dieter's lose-some, regain-more trap. You have already tried CBT if you have ever kept a food diary. Before my clients learn hypnosis, they track every morsel that passes their lips for a week or two. (You'll do the same in chapter 4, where you will find my food diary and other favorite CBT tools.) Raising awareness, every good hypnotherapist knows, is a key baby-step toward lasting change.

These two strategies, concludes a scientific re-analysis of eighteen studies, are far better than just one. Adding hypnosis to standard cognitive-behavioral therapy doubled the benefit of CBT, and those benefits *increased* substantially over time. That's right: all the study subjects lost weight during treatment, but in the most promising study, they kept on losing (and/or maintaining their goal weight) for up to two years after only a nine-week treatment.[5] In other words, hypnosis has been shown to facilitate weight loss *and* maintenance. Long-term!

Since you probably don't know that I use exclamation points like my Grammie's china—only on special occasions—you may not grasp the full significance of this finding. Considering that most dieters quickly regain what they lose and then some, it's nothing short of astounding. What's more, if the hypnotic suggestions are personalized and compassionate, a waist watcher's odds of success increase.

Having observed weight-loss clients for decades, I have learned to predict, without scientific instruments, imminent success. I do this by watching for a predictable phenomenon, a series of defining moments that I call "shifting to 'I can.'" I tell you about this phenomenon so you can watch for it in yourself. After some number of weeks, successes in the making start changing their tune: "I can't" lose weight becomes "maybe I can," which finally shifts to "I can." When this shift finally arrives, lighter days surely follow. Because this audible

Q I tried hypnosis once and it didn't work. Is it worth trying again?

A Absolutely. Especially if your first try was with a hypnotist who promised that, after a single session, you'd live slimly ever after. Many hypnotists have no advanced training or license to practice in their field of expertise. They may be "certified," but any manicurist or realtor can get "certified." Plus, a good number of hypnotists rely on standard trance scripts. The script may be well suited to one client, but not another. Apparent failures are often the result of a mismatch between subject and hypnotist.

precursor is the first hint of positive things to come, I listen for the moment "I can" divorces the "I can't" and all the heavy baggage that goes with that failed marriage. I listen for negativity to fade from the conversation. Because when waist watchers firm up their faith in their abilities, when they believe "Yes, I can!", they are well on their way. So when you notice this shift in your thoughts or conversation, see and believe it for what it really is—a sure sign of success. You *are* getting where you want to go.

One of the first clients to dramatically change her tune was Jill, a magazine editor whose flowing skirts and crossed arms could not hide the extra weight or heavy shame she carried. You name it, this discouraged dieter had tried it: Weight Watchers, Overeaters Anonymous, fen-phen. The sense of incompetence Jill had developed as a yo-yo dieter contrasted sharply with her considerable confidence as a respected editor and promising writer. She had always been able to lose weight, but it was only a matter of time before she would regain what she had lost, and then some. When her "then some" reached an all-time high of 275 pounds, she decided to take a less conventional route, a route that had delivered her mother out of migraine pain: hypnosis.

Jill was more realistic than most about the power of positive suggestion. Having witnessed her mom diligently practice self-hypnosis, she didn't expect overnight success. Week after week, Jill tapped into her considerable hypnotic talents and creative powers to rewrite her weight-loss script. If you could fast-forward through our work together, you could see Jill's can't-do attitude shift in an instant to "Wow, I really can!" You could witness her dramatic physical and mental transformation unfold before your eyes. Like Alice in Wonderland, you would see Jill get smaller and smaller, her chair seem to grow larger and larger. In a brief blur of time, you could marvel as more form-fitting fashions revealed what she had tried to hide under those flowing skirts: her waistline. You could witness this fortysomething lose and keep off some 50 pounds.

Over the course of three years, Jill would continue to feed herself positive suggestions and maintain a weight loss of more than 15 percent of her body weight, or about five sacks of potatoes. That's two sacks and two years more than the gold standard of long-term success as set by the National Weight Control Registry, a database of five thousand plus individuals who have maintained at least a 30-pound weight loss for one year.[6] In thirty-six months, you would see Jill regain nothing but confidence, enough confidence to tackle other elusive goals. She gained enough trust in her abilities to resurrect her lifelong dream of getting published. The talented editor wrote a series of personal essays, submitted them to literary magazines, and achieved her impossible dream: she finally got published. "When I get rid of the self-pity and do the math," she wrote in a personal essay, "I'm left with the ineluctable truth that if I take in fewer calories than I burn, I will lose the weight!" If the hypnotherapist were her personal editor, not her individual therapist, she might have suggested Jill say more about self-pity. She might have asked Jill to explain how, week after week, viewing herself through the therapist's compassionate eyes, Jill not only got rid of the self-pity, she got something invaluable: she got self-compassion.

A LITTLE HISTORY

To understand what's leading twenty-first-century waist watchers to this age-old practice, let's go back, back before obesity became a national epidemic, back before fat was declared a feminist issue, way back before "hypnosis" was considered a definable word by *Merriam Webster*, let alone a Google-able term. Depending on your viewpoint, hypnosis has been around since fire transfixed cavewomen, or at the very least, since an eighteenth-century Viennese doctor "mesmerized" clients back to health.

If you accept the idea of natural trance, that human beings naturally entrance themselves as needed, hypnosis was probably born with humanity. There's no shortage of evidence to make this case. Across time and space, historic texts describe trance phenomena—shamanic spells in primitive societies, curative "sleep" in Greece and Egypt, natural anesthesia induced by Indian yogis. One Biblical reference depicts an exceptional subject who can undergo surgery with hypnosis as the sole anesthetic: "And the Lord God caused a deep sleep to fall upon the man, and he slept; and he took one of his ribs, and closed up the place with flesh instead thereof." You didn't know Adam was highly hypnotizable? In Homer's Greek classic, *The Odyssey*, Odysseus entrances himself before treating a wound he sustained boar hunting: "And he stayed the black blood with a song of healing."

Sticklers for hard evidence will want to fast-forward to the late 1700s, when mesmerism inspired the first scientific inquiry into these ancient practices. Dressed to heal in his trademark purple flowing robes, Mesmer was a talented showman. With a magical pass of the hand, the flamboyant Viennese doctor caused curative convulsions and, voilà, the blind could see, the deathly ill could reclaim life. With a little help from his well-placed friends, Mesmer got great buzz, and it wasn't long before the doctor was "in" with the in crowd. Much as Oprah's approval launched Dr. Phil's career, raves from the likes of Mozart and his rich and famous contemporaries catapulted Mesmer's.

But Mesmer's popularity with the young, aristocratic lady clients raised one too many eyebrows, and yada yada yada, there was a royal inquiry. Another multitalented character, Ben Franklin, led the investigation into "animal magnetism," the universal healing force that Mesmer believed he was channeling. Does mesmerism work? That was the question Franklin's team set out to answer when they set up the first systematic study of what's now called hypnosis. Their conclusion sent a discredited Mesmer packing: animal magnetism doesn't exist; there's no such animal. Credit for the cure belonged to the client's imagination, not Mesmer's methods. But an interesting question remained: How exactly did clients imagine themselves well? The answer would have to wait.

But not the story, which forged on without a leading man. Interest in mesmerism persisted through the eventual name change, especially among doctors. If you're a fan of medical dramas, fast-forward to the next century when hypnosis proved indispensable on the battlefield for doing leg amputations and treating shell shock, later renamed post-traumatic stress disorder. Skip ahead another century, and suddenly health-care professionals are inducing trance in dental chairs, on operating tables, and on psychiatric couches, including one belonging to Dr. Sigmund Freud, who became infatuated with hypnosis, then disenchanted when his basic techniques delivered rapid results in only a few cases.[7] And before you know it, hypnosis was back in the doghouse, and didn't fully emerge again until science could validate Mesmer's claims.

Jump ahead to the late twentieth century, when the American Medical Association and other professional medical associations began to recognize hypnosis for what it is, a marvelous intervention for speeding recovery from outpatient surgery, easing chronic pain, diminishing gastrointestinal distress, reducing hot flashes and asthma attacks, and eradicating warts. Before you know it, leading psychological organizations, including the American Psychological Association, began to endorse hypnosis as a boon for the treatment of mental health issues, especially anxiety (phobias, panic disorder, generalized anxiety), post-traumatic stress, and habits (smoking, nail biting, hair pulling, and overeating).[8] And just like that, we have circled back to this day in history, back to right now.

So you see, it may have taken a couple of centuries for science to catch up with clinical experience, but once it did, hypnosis has proven to be an invaluable healing instrument for a range of health-care professionals, especially those who treat habits, anxiety, and other mind-body problems.

A MINI-TRANCE

When people ask me what's it like to get hypnotized for weight loss, I describe what it might feel like to gaze into the fireplace with a trusted friend who just happens to be a diet coach. It is relaxing yet focused work—and surprising in the magical way that sparks surprise.

For a better sense of the experience, read the next paragraph. Like the iconic swinging pocket-watch used in hypnosis, the italicized words are meant to focus your attention, deepen your relaxation, and open your mind. So sit back, make yourself comfortable, and take a few refreshing breaths. When you're ready for your first trance-lite experience, read the next paragraph. It will give you a preview of trance, not the full experience. And remember, you control the experience; you will only do what you choose to do.

Focusing all your attention on the italicized words, the crisp letters on the new page. So new. So promising. As you continue reading, you're opening your mind to the many interesting things that escape your everyday awareness: the light, comfortable weight of the book in your hands, for example. Notice your steady breathing rhythm: inhalations seamlessly shifting to exhalations, exhalations naturally leading to inhalations. As the rest of the world fades into the background now, your breathing slows, your facial expression softens, your shoulders relax. You are discovering how trance enhances your innate abilities and natural inclinations: your ability to focus, your receptiveness to encouraging words and positive suggestions for greater ease. Effortless change. You're seeing new possibilities, starting to imagine what it would be like to harness this careful attention, this single-minded focus on achieving that essential but elusive goal: a healthy, sustainable weight. Your true weight.

Even if your conscious mind harbors doubt, your unconscious mind holds the hope. The desire, the genuine desire to keep learning, discovering, to find your way.

Welcome back. Permit yourself to stretch, breathe, reorient to this typeface. Take another deep breath or two. If you have ever meditated, you might be wondering right about now, what's the difference between trance and meditation? Hypnosis and guided visualization? Excellent questions! Hypnosis and meditation are close cousins, with definite resemblances and real differences. Guided visualization is clearly related, but like the distant relative who shows up at big gatherings, it's hard to say exactly how. Visualizations are often meditations or trances that have been simplified or otherwise altered for mass appeal. To keep the comparison simple, I will concentrate on meditation.

A DEEP RELAXATION

Both hypnosis and meditation are remarkably portable, and therefore quite accommodating to busy schedules, travel plans, and other real-life challenges. Even if you are overextended and sleep-deprived, there's always room for a five-minute meditation or trance. Both practices can be relaxing, yet relaxation is neither a prerequisite nor the inevitable result of either. Mindful awareness and trance can invite a deep physiological relaxation that measurably alters heart rate, body temperature, and muscle tension. Both can initially inspire more than a little uneasiness, especially among new practitioners. Novice meditators and hypnotic subjects inadvertently conjure feelings of inadequacy and other less-than-tender feelings when they criticize themselves for doing "it" (the practice) wrong. In both cases, relaxation comes from staying with "it," learning to go with the flow without judgment.

Traditionally, practitioners sit or lie down with closed eyes, but it's not uncommon to meditate or undergo trance with eyes wide open, standing, or walking. It's even possible, researchers have shown, to go into trance while riding a stationary bicycle. However you choose to practice meditation or hypnosis—and practice is a must—know that all practitioners are not created equal. All the motivation in the world can't make up for natural ability. The exceptions—the Dalai Lama, the birthing mother who undergoes a C-section sans anesthesia—are truly exceptional.

The big difference between the two practices is what you do, or don't do. In hypnosis, it's all about "doing": active problem-solving with a goal of effecting change. And yet, both can and do bring about positive change. In meditation, it's more about "being," accepting what is, changing nothing. Another good-sized difference is how beginners respond. Despite worries of doing "it" wrong, new hypnotic subjects usually have an easier, happier time of it than first-time meditators, who commonly complain of anxiety, boredom, pain, or feeling "spaced-out."[9] In trance, the power of the mind is focused with suggestions; in meditation, the mind's content gets little attention. For responsive hypnotic subjects, simple suggestions can do what weeks of meditative practice cannot.

Nowhere is the difference more striking than in the Stroop Test, a mental challenge popular with psychology researchers and Internet surfers. In the Stroop Test, subjects are given the name of a color in a different colored ink, and then have to identify the ink color, not the word. For example, the ink color might be red, but the text will say the word "blue." While six weeks of meditation practice had little effect on the Stroop Effect (the delayed reaction caused by the color confusion), hypnotic suggestion virtually eliminated it.[10]

Similarly, hypnotic slimming suggestions have a dramatic effect. Separate studies have shown both hypnosis and meditation to be reliable ways of getting a handle on everyday eating disturbances (compulsive overeating, yo-yo dieting) and eating disorders (bulimia, binge-eating disorder), but researchers have yet to compare the two as slimming strategies.[11] The lone researcher who combined the two practices—blended meditative principles with weight-loss suggestions—got the most dramatic, longest-lasting results.[12]

FINDING THINSPIRATION

Feast on Food Films

Dieters are trapped in no-win arguments with themselves. The one-sided argument goes something like this: "My problem is I enjoy eating too much. If I let myself enjoy more, I'll eat more. If I eat more, I'll gain more." Sound familiar? In this mindset, it's unimportant if French women don't get fat slathering baguettes with butter; you do just thinking about dry toast. If you want to lose weight, you'll have to deny yourself your favorite foods.

So you say until along comes a movie that celebrates eating, and the iron grip of this illogical logic loosens for a few hours. Munching popcorn under the cover of darkness, you feast your eyes on the Technicolor smorgasbord. You remember the simple, sensual pleasures of dining with friends and family. You subliminally entertain the possibility of eating without food restrictions, living like those slender characters on screen: diet-free.

Thanks to DVDs and DVRs, you don't have to wait for the next uplifting food flick to come to a Cineplex near you. Throw yourself a movie festival and uplift yourself with a feature film, such as *Julie & Julia* or *Like Water for Chocolate*; a mindful-eating documentary, like *How to Cook for Your Life*; or a single scene that elevates one bite into a sensual feast as *Tess* does with a strawberry. Hit the play button and just savor.

In my own practice, I have also found this best-of-both-worlds approach to make a dramatic difference. When I started adding mindful-eating suggestions based on meditative techniques into the hypnotic mix, my weight-loss clients found themselves automatically eating with greater awareness of hunger and fullness signals, and easily losing weight. You have already met one such client: Katherine.

A DIETER'S FABLE

Remember Katherine, the Snickers-chomping grandmother who lost 15 pounds in twelve weeks? I tell you the next chapter of her weight-loss story because Katherine's story is every dieter's story. Because this second chapter tells it like it really is; because it discourages and encourages, discourages fairy-tale fantasies, encourages genuine hope. Because it's a modern-day fable with a timeless moral that will help you write a new, more promising beginning to the rest of your weight-loss story.

Here it is: Happily lighter after three months of weekly therapy, Katherine felt ready to spread her wings and fly solo. She wasn't worried. My return policy (more sessions as needed) felt like enough of a safety net. She promised to stay in touch, which she did: "I wanted to let you know that my doctor was really impressed with my weight loss," she e-mailed. "Thank you so much!" Five months would pass before her blue eyes would brighten my doorway again. In the seven steps around the little blue coffee table to my couch, her rounder face and fuller hips tipped me off to the reason for her return visit. She had thoroughly enjoyed her travels, especially visiting the grandchildren, but, no surprise, frequent flying and restaurant dining had waylaid her best intentions. What surprised us both was how Katherine felt about regaining half of what she had lost: she felt rather encouraged.

"When I'd regain weight in the past," she said, "I'd feel so hopeless. There was nothing I could do." But this time was different. Because she knew exactly what to do, it wasn't hard to reclaim a sense of self-efficacy and confidence. Listening to Katherine was like hearing myself talk: "Getting back on track is as easy as getting back to the basics," she said. "Food logs, self-hypnosis, mindful eating, loving-kindness." By session's end, Katherine was clear. More than hypnotherapy sessions, all she really needed to renew motivation was a new hypnosis CD.

The moral of Katherine's story is a quirky T-shirt slogan: "Rewrite your script." If you really want a happier ending to your tired old weight-loss story, keep rewriting until you get it right. Rewrite your inner monologue. Rather than mentally rehashing the same despairing

message—"I'll always eat like a pig!"—write a more empowering
self-suggestion: "More and more, I am savoring delicious, nutritious
food." Alter your plot in some small but significant way—send yourself on a beach vacation, and let the sound of the mesmerizing waves
carry you into a deep relaxation. Adopt a kinder, gentler attitude; try
a new, diet-free weight-loss strategy; find a supporting character to
supply hope and motivation—a living, breathing hypnotherapist or
a self-hypnosis audio or video companion. Keep changing the action,
the setting, the cast, until your heroine triumphs. Until your leading
lady, *you,* gets where she's going.

Great idea, but how do you draft a better script? Fire your scriptwriter? Sure, Bill Murray finally finds his way out of *Groundhog Day,*
but his scriptwriter was brilliant. If you could have fired your scriptwriter, you would have. The hack who wrote your original screenplay
only made you heavier in THE END.

Fortunately, the script doctor is in. The rewrite will be easier than
you think, given that the script doctor just so happens to be a hypnotherapist with no shortage of excellent suggestions. Here's one: take
a deep, refreshing inhalation, a long slooooooooooooooooooow exhalation, and those heavy self-doubts, set 'em aside. You'll feel lighter.
One more thing: when you reread the opening scene of your inspired
script revision, the desperate character in search of a better diet will
look only vaguely familiar, like someone you knew from grade school
or summer camp.

WINNING WEIGHT-LOSS SUGGESTIONS FOR STAYING SLIM

Eat food. Not too much. Mostly plants.

MICHAEL POLLAN

If you have opened directly to this chapter, it might be news to you that hypnosis, the age-old, all-purpose therapeutic tool, promotes lasting weight loss without dieting. If you have gotten chapter 3 under your belt, you already know that positive suggestion has the power to help waist watchers lose and maintain weight after only a brief course of hypnotherapy. And even if you are aware that most people are somewhat hypnotizable, and that research has shown fat-fearing women to be particularly hypnotizable, you are probably still wondering: Will it work for me?

Chapter 4 will, first and foremost, help you answer that question—help you assess your hypnotic ability so you can determine the best way to integrate hypnosis into your weight-loss program. Once you have assessed your hypnotizability level, you can then begin to incorporate the hypnotic suggestions that follow as you see fit. (Even if you're not all that hypnotizable, these suggestions can help you consciously take charge of your eating.) In between, you can learn everything you need to know about self-hypnosis, and a little more about cognitive-behavioral therapy (CBT). The CBT tools you will acquire will help you personalize the hypnotic suggestions for your best and easiest shot at sustainable weight loss. Along the way, you will take a hypnotic-responsiveness quiz, set up goals and a progress graph, begin a food log, and learn to hypnotize yourself. If you try self-hypnosis and really like it, you will want to keep at it, practicing until you reach your goals or as long as you find it helpful.

NO STUPID QUESTIONS

Q I'm afraid I won't be a good hypnotic subject, but I really want to get hypnotized. Can motivation make me more responsive to hypnotic suggestions?

A High motivation is a great quality in a hypnotic subject. Even if you have low hypnotic ability, if you are highly motivated to practice self-hypnosis, you can do exceptionally well. Conversely, if you have exceptional abilities, but zero motivation, well, don't expect much, unless of course you are willing to explore motivational issues in hypnotherapy.

So first, back to that pressing question: How will hypnosis work for you? You can answer that question two simple ways: (1) Call your friendly neighborhood hypnotherapist for a formal hypnotic assessment, or (2) Skip the formalities and the expense, and play twenty-one questions. Twenty-one is the number of questions you will answer on Jean's Hypnotic-Responsiveness Quiz, the home version of a standardized measure called the Tellegen Absorption Scale, which measures openness to absorbing experiences as well as self-perception-altering experiences.[1] Absorbing experiences are everyday occurrences, like losing yourself in a good book. Alterations in self-perception may feel more unusual, but they're not uncommon. You've had a self-altering experience if you've suddenly felt school-aged at a class reunion. My quiz assesses the same traits as the research tool, but takes into account the experiences of waist watchers.

Like the self-compassion quiz in chapter 1, it's important to remember why you're putting yourself to the test. In this case, you're assessing whether the route you're studying—currently hypnosis—is one you might like to explore on your weight-loss journey. And if it is, discovering what's the best way for you to travel this enchanting territory. Answer each question as honestly as you can.

QUIZ 2
Jean's Hypnotic-Responsiveness Quiz

If you can daydream, chances are you can benefit from hypnosis. And I have yet to meet someone who doesn't daydream. But a better predictor of your hypnotic responsiveness is what psychotherapists call "mental absorption," the ability to tune out the outside world, tune in to the inner mind. Daydreaming is one aspect of absorption, but there are others. Answer these twenty-one yes-or-no questions to assess your absorption, and predict where you fall on the hypnotic-responsiveness scale. Choose "yes" for always, sometimes, occasionally, or kind of. And check "no" for never, not usually, infrequently, probably not, or definitely not.

Have you ever:

☒Yes ☐No   1. Momentarily felt like a big kid, behaving or reacting as if you were your younger self?

☒Yes ☐No   2. Zoned out while eating junk food, mall shopping, Internet surfing?

☒Yes ☐No   3. Gotten so engrossed in a good movie, TV show, or book that it was as if you were transported out of your world—your body and surroundings—and into a character's?

☒Yes ☐No   4. Driven somewhere as if on autopilot? Or gazed out the bus window only to "wake up" suddenly at your stop?

☒Yes ☐No   5. Played a sport, a musical instrument, or written

something almost automatically, with more ease
and grace than you could have deliberately?

☒Yes ☐No 6. Experienced a mystical experience, or what many
call an "out-of-body experience"?

☐Yes ☒No 7. Dwelled on weight gain and/or imagined you'd
gotten so heavy, it felt difficult, if not impossible,
to move?

☒Yes ☐No 8. Ignited your imagination by focusing on the snap,
crackle, and pop of a wood fire?

☒Yes ☐No 9. Noticed that you think in images more
than words?

☒Yes ☐No 10. Shifted out of your usual state into a very different
experience of yourself?

☐Yes ☒No 11. Sensed someone's presence before you were close
enough to see or hear the person?

☒Yes ☐No 12. Washed the dishes or finished some other
everyday task thinking about something
completely different?

☒Yes ☐No 13. Remembered something way back when so vividly
that it felt as if you were experiencing it in the here
and now?

☒Yes ☐No 14. Delighted in life's little pleasures: blowing soap
bubbles, gazing into your lover's eyes, playing
water glasses like a xylophone?

☒Yes ☐No 15. Noticed how certain smells, like freshly baked
cookies, evoke vivid memories or take you back to
earlier experiences?

☒Yes ☐No 16. Felt that your body continued experiencing
something even after you stopped experiencing it;
for example, feeling like you were still at sea after
coming ashore?

☒Yes ☐No   17. Been enthralled by the sound of a voice or the turn
of a phrase?

☐Yes ☒No   18. Smelled a color, heard a texture, or experienced
one sense as another?

☐Yes ☒No   19. Discovered music in what others only perceive
as noise?

☐Yes ☒No   20. Turned away from the mirror, but the image
lingered, almost as if you were still gazing at
your reflection?

☒Yes ☐No   21. Been deeply moved by a thunderstorm or rainbow?

Scoring Sheet

Give yourself 1 point for every "yes" answer.

Total Score: __16__   Date: __11__ / __27__ / __11__

Your Score and What to Make of It

When it comes to hypnotizability, 0–7 suggests you are on the low
end of the spectrum, but with a few adjustments, hypnosis can still
be a powerful tool for reshaping your eating habits and your waistline
—in your case, the suggestions will work best when you consciously
repeat them like positive affirmations rather than counting on your
unconscious mind to retain them; 8–15, you have ample hypnotic
ability, or moderate hypnotizability, which is just one good reason
to seriously consider exploring hypnosis for weight loss; 16–21, you
have exceptional ability, lucky you. Because you are on the high end
of the spectrum, losing weight can be so much easier!

THE POWER TOOLS

Independently, hypnosis and cognitive-behavioral therapy (CBT)
are powerful weight-loss strategies. Together, they are superpowered.

Because CBT is a great way to set weight-loss goals and track progress, not to mention problem-solve, clients typically pick up a few good CBT tools before they learn self-hypnosis techniques. Not only are these easy-to-use tools a handy way to jump-start weight loss, they are great for maintaining your new way of being, week after week, month after month. Once you get to your desired weight, they are just as handy for weight maintenance. They are especially handy for low-hypnotizable subjects, who reliably benefit from conscious strategies like these tools.

I call them Power Tools because, well, they're powerful and therefore require careful handling. Without fair warning, too many dieters inadvertently turn these tools on themselves as weapons of self-criticism. If you have ever tried using any of the tools contained in this section, you know how easy it is to judge yourself harshly for a second helping of mashed potatoes, another spoonful of ice cream—especially if you have enlisted a less-than-compassionate therapist or diet coach with hypercritical eyes. Even with fair warning and good intentions, harsh criticism is almost inevitable. If, or should I say when, you catch yourself wielding one of these therapeutic tools as a weapon, pause and remember: *handle with care.*

The first tool you will learn how to handle with self-compassion is the Attainable Goal List. Once you have set realistic goals for yourself, the Food Log will help you detect and correct problematic eating patterns, and the Progress Graph will help you mindfully track weight trends (the losses and the gains). If the possibility of weight gain on the way to permanent weight loss inspires undue concern, pause and remember: *handle with care.* How? That's what you are about to learn.

THINK SELF-KIND THOUGHTS

Your Inner Critic:

I really blew it this week; I'm sure I gained _____ *(fill in the metaphorical amount of weight you fear you gained).*

Your Compassionate Response:

_____

_____

_____

_____

TOOL 1
Attainable Goal List

To begin, you need a set of *attainable* goals that can not only be attained, but maintained. I underscore "attainable" because your success depends on it. Setting your sights beyond your reach invites failure. If you have ever counted carbs, calories, or some such dietary measure, you have courted enough failure. You would like to meet success. But how? You can't advertise for your dream weight. Or can you? Setting attainable goals is kind of like writing a personal ad for a slimmer you. Don't wait for success to find you: roll out the welcome mat. Set both measurable and immeasurable goals in attainable increments so you will recognize success early and invite it to stay.

A measurable goal (think body weight) can be observed and quantified. Immeasurable goals, such as feeling more attractive or energetic, are obviously harder to measure. For measurable goals, you will need to set your sights on a unit of measurement that is within reach—and a wide target range always helps too. If pounds lost and gained have the power to make or break your day, consider choosing a more neutral measure, like waist circumference or clothing size, or adjusting your attitude toward your weight. (If you want to learn how to take a self-compassionate stance on the bathroom scale, be sure to take this chapter's Personal Slimming Lesson.) Also forget about hitting a tiny bull's-eye, and take aim at three broad categories: "enviable," "realistic," and "bearable." Recognize your ideal, to-die-for weight; your circumference or size as "enviable" and not all that attainable; and then reset your sights on "realistic," a number you can reach without starving or exhausting yourself. Better yet, aim first for "bearable," the least thrilling but most attainable of the three categories.

Envisioning an "enviable" goal is a no-brainer. Undoubtedly you have had this to-die-for number in mind for quite some time. To determine what's "realistic" now, consider measures you have used in previous weight-loss efforts as well as current recommendations from medical professionals, personal trainers, and health organizations in league with the American Heart Association. Your "bearable" goal might be a number you would have dismissed in your youth, like the nerd who asked you to the prom. But given your age, health, abilities, and the fact that what's bearable now offers many of the same health benefits as what's realistic, it's become less objectionable, more appealing. Expand your measurable goal list by adding quantifiable health benefits, including measures of fitness (resting heart rate, walking or running mph), physical health (blood pressure, sugar and cholesterol levels), and mental health (stress level, binge frequency).[2]

PERSONAL SLIMMING LESSON

Scale: Friend or Foe?

Many waist watchers see the scale as an important key to lasting weight loss, but what's your view? Has weighing in done more to open or lock your door to sustainable slimness? If you're convinced that regularly stepping on the scale eventually pushes you off the weight-loss wagon, you would likely do better with a more neutral measure (a tape measure, fat caliper, clothing size).

If your jury's still out on weighing in, weigh the evidence. Consider if the scale has hindered past slimming efforts. If it's proved a hindrance, think about when that was, where you were in life, how you approached the scale. To consider if the scale has proven helpful, follow the same line of questioning. If you can, remember the specifics: Did you weigh in publicly or privately? Was your attitude more objective or reactive? The embodiment of loving-kindness or tough love? Clients who consider the scale more friend than foe approach it with a mix of objectivity and self-compassion—objectivity for assessing weight trends, self-compassion for addressing emotional reactions to less-than-favorable trends.

Before you reach your verdict, you may find you need more evidence. If that's your case, practice taking a kinder stance on the bathroom scale. Whether you gain or lose, deepen your breathing and meditate on loving-kindness: "May I be safe, healthy, happy, at ease." Then objectively review what you have eaten since the last weigh-in, making connections when you can between your nutritional intake and the digital readout. Over time, notice if a kinder, more objective viewpoint improves your relationship with the scale. Collect as much evidence as you need in order to close this case.

Immeasurable goals may defy measurement, but not observation. You don't need a scale or some other tool to let you know that you have reached one of these less measurable goals. If you are like most waist watchers, you just know it, which is why immeasurable goals don't need to be broken down into mini-goals. But for those who fail to see or feel the immeasurable difference that weight loss makes, measurable goals can be especially validating.

The most common goals of the immeasurable type involve feeling *more* (attractive, energetic, confident, at peace with food) and *less* (self-conscious, self-critical, obsessed with food). Less common, but equally valuable, are goals of greater acceptance (of your sweet tooth, your imperfect shape, your clothing size). Immeasurable goals require looking ahead, but it's worth looking back on those activities or interactions that contributed to previous weight-loss successes.

Thinking about goals is all well and good, but making a written commitment to yourself is way better. Signing your Jane Hancock to a personal contract is your way of declaring that you mean business. If deadlines motivate you, give yourself one or several, or identify shorter- and longer-term goals. Whatever your timetable, grab paper and pen, and write them down.

Measurable Goals

Enviable: _____

Realistic: _____

Bearable: _____

_____

Immeasurable Goals

_____

_____

_____

Signature: _____   Date: _____ / _____ / _____

Review your goals on occasion or at regular intervals (monthly, quarterly, and annually). When you reach a goal, celebrate if you like, but keep the list going by updating, adding, and modifying as you go along.

TOOL 2
Food Logs

Because it's such a portable and powerful tool, you have probably used a food log at some point in your dieting career. Hard to believe that writing down everything you eat makes much difference, but according to one of the largest weight-loss studies ever, it makes a big difference. Study subjects who faithfully recorded every morsel that passed their lips lost twice as much weight as their less faithful cohorts. Those who couldn't be bothered still lost weight—about nine pounds in six months—but those who kept at least six daily logs a week lost 18 pounds in half a year.[3] If all you got for your food-logging efforts was shame and weight gain, it *is* hard to believe that keeping a food log could make any positive difference. Unless, of course, you take a different, more self-compassionate approach to this standard-issue slimming tool.

In theory, food logs work because they give you pause, pause to notice how you feel (hungry, angry, lonely?) and what you need (a snack, a hug, a nap?), and pause to identify and correct problematic eating patterns. In other words, they help you become more mindful of what you are eating. In practice, as I have mentioned, food logs can also backfire. When viewed with a critical eye, a record of your caloric intake can actually inspire overeating. To reap the benefits without the detriments, adopt my motto: handle with care. Review your food log with self-compassionate eyes.

On the following page is a sample chart my clients keep, and I recommend you keep it for at least one to two weeks, or as long as you

FOOD LOG

Day: Date:

Time	Food & Drink Consumed	x	Place	Hunger*	Essay: Thoughts, Feelings, Situation

Put x next to food or drink that you view as excessive.
*Degree of Hunger: 0 = not hungry 1 = slightly hungry 2 = somewhat hungry 3 = very hungry

find it helpful. Fill out one chart a day, making entries ASAP after each meal and snack so you don't forget anything.

My log is fairly self-explanatory, but it's worth reviewing the columns. In the Time column, record *when* you ate. Under Food and Drink Consumed, describe *what* you ate, guesstimating quantities. (No need to weigh and measure.) If what you consumed seemed excessive (portions, calories, etc.) put an *x* next to it. Under Place, record *where* you ate. Rate your Hunger level before you ate, using the four-point scale at the bottom of the log. And under Essay, note anything (thoughts, feelings, situation) that positively or negatively influenced your eating experience.

When you have amassed a week of logs, put on your food-detective cap and investigate the patterns that encouraged and discouraged healthy eating. In tracking healthful patterns, keep in mind food writer Michael Pollan's pithy prescription: "Eat food. Not too much. Mostly plants."[4] Let me elaborate: Eat meals and snacks that feature a variety of nutritious, delicious real foods to the point of comfortable fullness. Fill your plate with more food from plants (fruits, vegetables, whole-grain bread, brown rice, beans and other legumes, heart-healthy fats), less from animals (meats—keep them lean; dairy—stick to lowfat). To eat more healthfully, you don't have to go so far as to become a vegetarian or a teetotaler. But if you enjoy meat and alcohol, do keep your consumption modest, especially if you are going for sustainable weight loss.

It's easy to spot problematic patterns if you look for the polar opposite of Pollan's prescription in the Food and Drink Consumed column: supersized portions of meat, dairy, and high-calorie, well-preserved processed foods. More elusive is the likeliest suspect to inspire such choices: undereating. As counterintuitive as it sounds, eating too little is a physiological setup for eating too much. Even if you are convinced that you eat too much, not too little, watch for undereating's many wily guises: puny "dieter's" portions, missing food groups, missing meals, long stretches between meals, wild-eyed hunger. Other common setups: tasteless low-cal entrees, monotonous food choices, "diet" food and drinks, megadoses of caffeine and sugar substitutes. Search the Place and Essay columns for clues to emotional eating—the locations, situations, thoughts, and feelings that trigger overeating. But keep in mind: until you start feeding yourself a steady diet of nutritious, delicious food, it's tough to tell the difference between emotional and physiological overeating.

FINDING THINSPIRATION

Delight Your Palate

There's nothing inspiring about a boring menu plan. Even if your daily menus used to please your palate, it's worth noticing if that's still the case. Taste buds are happy to support your slimming efforts . . . if you serve them a variety of delicious, nutritious food. But bore them day after day after day, and they will demand treats that are exceedingly delicious, but not particularly nutritious.

Keep yourself and your palate thinspired by spicing up old menus with healthy new recipes. Find time to go to the bookstore and find healthy cookbooks that inspire and delight you. Surf the Internet for favorite recipes from health-conscious cooks at popular health spas and whole-food restaurants. If you have no time to cook, don't worry; buy takeout. Between hither and yon, pick up a quick, tasty bite at a natural foods store, farmers market, or gourmet shop. Do yourself a mutual favor—keep delighting your taste buds, and they will happily get behind your weight-loss plan.

Now you are ready for a practice investigation. On the following page is a food log from Heidi, an inspiring client you will meet in chapter 5.

Heidi started that Monday with such good intentions: whole grains, lean protein, fruits and vegetables. But she set herself up for overeating by undereating. Her skimpy daytime intake fueled her nighttime mini-binge. Did you spot other suspect patterns: monotonous choices; missing meals; long stretches between eating; lots of processed food, caffeine, and artificial sweetener? You will sharpen your investigation skills with practice, but you get the idea.

FOOD LOG
Day: Monday   Date: 6/8

Time	Food & Drink Consumed	x	Place	Hunger*	Essay: Thoughts, Feelings, Situation
7 a.m.	large latte w/ 2 pkgs NutraSweet		car	0	I ate too much last night. I can't eat breakfast.
10 a.m.	chocolate PowerBar		desk	3	Yum, I'm starving!
2 p.m.	multigrain sub roll, turkey, lettuce, tomato 16 oz. Diet Coke whole-grain Fig Newton		desk	2	Healthy lunch! Feels good
4:30 p.m.	12 grapes 16 oz. Diet Coke		desk	2	I'm tired.
7 p.m.	multigrain sub roll, turkey, lettuce, tomato whole-grain Fig Newton		den	3	I don't feel like cooking dinner. I guess I'll have lunch again.
9 p.m.	1/2 cup frozen yogurt 10 whole-grain crackers 10 mixed nuts 3 jelly donuts	x	den	3	I was so good all day, but now I have no control!

Put x next to food or drink that you view as excessive.
*Degree of Hunger: 0 = not hungry 1 = slightly hungry 2 = somewhat hungry 3 = very hungry

If you want a full-sized, blank food log, visit the Resources page on my website (jeanfain.com). Or create your own on a computer spreadsheet or old-fashioned graph paper. Still got that pen?

TOOL 3
Progress Graphs

Last but not least: every compassionate weight-loss toolbox needs a progress graph. Used consistently, a self-monitoring tool like this graph is an important key to lasting success, according to the overwhelming majority of the individuals in the National Weight Control Registry, those waist watchers who have kept off 30-plus pounds for at least a year.

Most members equipped themselves with a scale for weekly, if not daily, weigh-ins, but that doesn't mean you have to follow the pack.

You can use any reliable measure (waist circumference, body-fat percentage, clothing size), as long as you use it on a regular schedule. That schedule is your call, too. Some clients wouldn't think of starting the day without hopping on the scale; others find daily weight fluctuations unsettling and prefer weighing in weekly, instead gauging their day-to-day progress by observing the positive, immeasurable changes (mood, energy, sense of well-being, etc.).

Like food logs, progress graphs offer greater awareness of positive and negative trends, and therefore offer greater choice about when to persist and when to take corrective action. If you are making progress, notice what's helping you progress, and keep on doing it. It was as simple as that for Katherine, the successful, self-compassionate dieter you met in the first chapter. Take a look at her graph below.

No one welcomes word of weight gain, but if viewed as news you can use, a negative trend is useful information, a compelling reason to resurrect healthy habits. As soon as you notice that you are heading

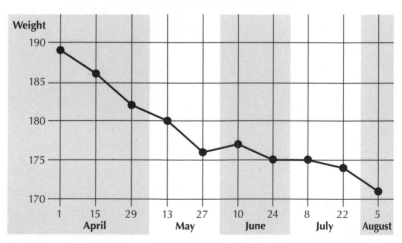

KATHERINE'S WEIGHT GRAPH

in the wrong direction, ask yourself: What were you doing when you were making good progress? When did progress become regress: the holidays, your birthday, the day your gym membership expired? What simple steps can you take to get back on track? Should you get back to food logs, the gym, self-compassion practice?

Now is a good time to choose a measure and a self-measurement schedule. (If you decide your measure is more demoralizing than motivating, try another, or change the measuring schedule.) It's also a good time to get out the graph paper and make a Progress Graph. It's so simple even a math-phobe can do it: Just draw a horizontal and vertical axis—one line across the bottom of the page, one along the left edge. At regular intervals, mark the date on the horizontal axis, your measurement on the vertical. To gain momentum from positive trends and to stay on top of negative ones, break your measure into small increments: single pounds, inches, clothing sizes. My weight graph measures pounds in five-pound blocks, big enough to add hatch marks for individual pounds, even ounces.

Leave room on your graph for the possibility of weight gain. In the off chance that your weight goes up before it goes down, know that you've got company. Some waist watchers get going that way. Also make space for notes about vacations, illnesses, and other circumstances that can help you make sense of the trends. Finally, if graphs overwhelm you with anxiety, find a friend, roommate, or partner to help you set it up and fill it out. Or at least, a pencil with a fresh eraser.

WINNING WEIGHT-LOSS SUGGESTIONS

Finally, the pièce de résistance: hypnosis. You are about to learn six easy hypnotic practices; I like to think of them as recipes for healthy slimness. Follow the instructions, and you will first calm your body and open your mind, then feed your receptive unconscious some lasting, slimming suggestions that will make it easier, if not effortless, to eat healthfully and lose weight.

Not to worry, you don't need elaborate training or fancy equipment. But you do need a willingness to formalize what has been informal until now—trance, that dreamy but focused state of attention—and the readiness to feed yourself a steady diet of suggestions that are positive, personalized, and compassionate. There won't be any negative, generic, and cruel directives like the ones tele-hypnotists have been known to give unsuspecting subjects, like "Cheeseburgers will taste like worms" or "Cookies will sicken you." Their effect is, at best, temporary. My recipes are not only positive, they're quick and easy, requiring only minimal preparation. If you've tried other practices in this book, you will find the preparations quite similar, but somewhat different.

Ready: Hypnosis takes time, about fifteen to twenty minutes a day. Many hypnotherapists suggest one long daily trance, but they are probably unfamiliar with the very successful hypnotic weight-loss study where subjects lost more weight and kept it off longer by doing three short trances before three square meals a day. Truth be told: my clients have lost weight doing shorter and longer trances whenever they please.

The trances you are about to learn are short (about five minutes), sweet, and flexible. If you want a deeper, more relaxing experience, do two or three trances in one sitting. If you would rather do a series of five-minute trances throughout the day, you won't go as deep, but you will keep the suggestions fresh in mind. If you have only time for one trance, do one. More is better, but one beats none.

Set: Hypnosis also takes space—a safe, quiet place where you can sit or lie back comfortably. If your chosen seating arrangement proves uncomfortable, choose again. Do what you can ahead of time to prevent distractions—and to incorporate those that are inevitable into your trance. If, for example, you are imagining a cloudless, blue sky and you hear honking horns, embellish the sky image with a flock of geese, flying in perfect V-formation. If you can't work *with* the distraction, view it as an invitation to pay attention.

If it comes to your attention that you're sleepy, consider practicing at a more alert time or taking a more upright position, if not a nap. Trance works best when you are awake, relaxed, yet focused enough to follow the script and deal with a pressing matter if one were to arise. But play it safe: don't multitask. Don't trance and drive, for example, or simultaneously do any activity that needs full attention.

Trance: If you have ever tried hypnosis, you probably closed your eyes and let the hypnotherapist guide you. For the upcoming hypnotic practices, you will need to keep your eyes open and follow the scripts verbatim, at least to start. Rather than just reading the words, invite a fuller experience by bringing the suggestions to life with your senses. Imagine seeing, feeling, touching, hearing, even tasting what's suggested.

Once you have mastered the basic steps of trance, if not learned the scripts by heart, feel free to close your eyes and go deeper into the experience. If you've got *The Self-Compassion Diet* audio, you can let my mesmerizing voice guide you. Otherwise, consider enlisting a willing reader, preferably someone with a soothing voice, or recording your own reading voice.

Every practice is a complete hypnotic experience, guiding you in, around, and out of trance. The practice scripts share the same structure, but like pizza, no two are alike. In fact, the same script can engender different experiences at different times. Also, different people can have very different experiences with the same script. So it's important to go with the flow of actual experience. Just as important, set aside all expectations but the following one: with every trance, expect to follow the same six steps—Focus, Breathe, Suggest, Post-It, Return, Reflect.

Let me explain: Focus fixes the attention, signaling mind and body that it's trance time. Breathe guides you into relaxation and your inner experience. Suggest is the most important piece—the suggestions for healthy slimness—which you individualize by adding goals and other personal specifics. Post-it, or post-hypnotic suggestion, is the piece that sticks in your mind after you come out of trance. Return brings you back to present experience and full alertness. Reflect—the last, but no less important, step—gives you a chance to look back before rushing off into your busy life; it allows for a quiet moment to notice thoughts, feelings, insights, or whatever came up for you during trance. A good way to hold on to important reflections is to commit them to paper or your journal.

Try all the scripts as they are written in this book, and then take creative license if you feel compelled to do so. Create new trances by mixing and matching favorite steps from the various scripts. For example, record Focus from the first script, Breathe from the second, Suggest from the third, and so on. Or keep trance fresh by staying tuned to my website for updates on new recordings. Try it, see if you like it.

PRACTICE 7
Outstanding Suggestions

Ever wish you craved delicious, nutritious food more than salty, fatty, sugary

NO STUPID QUESTIONS

Q I've listened to a lot of hypnosis CDs, and I can't help but wonder: Why do so many hypnotists talk as if English is their second language? They're often grammatically incorrect, indirect, if not confusing. And they tend to repeat themselves. What's up with that?

A You're right! The language of hypnosis has its own rhyme and reason. Like all languages, there are different dialects, such as Ericksonian hypnosis, which may be the most distinctive and confusing.

But, by and large, hypnotists talk like foreigners because they are speaking directly to the unconscious mind, which is generally more receptive to suggestions that are indirect, rhythmic, repetitive, and playful. Hypnotists are more like poets than prose writers—they may adhere to certain structural guidelines, but they often take liberties with sentence structure.

treats? Do you realize you have the power to grant yourself that wish? Open your mind to these outstanding suggestions inspired by the very best hypnotic weight-loss study.[5]

Focus: Make yourself comfortable, let your breathing naturally deepen, and focus your attention on reading. That's right, as you narrow your focus to the printed word, you can't help but notice the letters changing before your eyes.

Breathe: And as you enjoy the subtle shifts in color, shape, and light, you're remembering to breathe, comfortably and naturally. Naturally and comfortably. On the next in-breath, take a deep full breath and hold it. Pause in silence for five seconds. As you let your breath out, let it all the way out, and feel yourself floating down, down, deep . . . into a very relaxing, quiet, receptive state.

Suggest: Now pay close attention: more and more, you are drawn to delicious, nutritious foods, especially local, seasonal, farm-fresh fare. Automatically, effortlessly, you are eating more mindfully, savoring each bite. Eating more slowly . . . with more satisfaction. Appreciating food's color, taste, and texture. In giving yourself permission to eat what you want, to eat satisfying portions from all the food groups, you are feeling more confident, in your ability to eat when you're hungry and stop when you're full. The more you pay attention to when your tummy is comfortably full and your taste buds are happily satisfied, the more you can trust your body's signals that it is nourished.

Increasingly, nourishing yourself appeals more than depriving yourself.

Attending to the signals of physical hunger, noticing how they differ from the sensations of emotional desires, you are better able to tend to whatever needs attending.

Post-It: To your happy surprise, you are progressing, slowly but surely, toward a healthy, sustainable weight. You are feeling more attractive, energetic, confident. [You can add your personal goals here.] You are living a fuller, more satisfying life.

Return: Now, as you refocus on taking deep, satisfying breaths, breathing slowly, quietly, rhythmically, it's only natural to return to normal alertness, to the present moment, feeling very relaxed, refreshed, and alert.

Reflect: What lingers? Notice lasting images, lingering phrases, palpable feelings. Make a mental note, if not a journal entry, of whatever seems most noteworthy.

PRACTICE 8
Encouraging Words[6]

Practicing this simple trance before meals helps you stop and smell, taste, and appreciate what you are about to eat. Whatever your hypnotic ability, another option is to repeat these encouraging words at bedtime, when the mind is especially suggestible. You will most likely wake up feeling more in control of your eating.

Focus: Settle in to a comfortable position; focus your attention on the printed page and the rhythmic breath. Natural, comfortable breaths. Comfortable, natural breaths. On the in-breath, taking a full four seconds to inflate the tummy like a balloon, on the out-breath, giving yourself eight long seconds to slowly, gradually deflate it. Inhaling, exhaling, focusing on the breath.

Breathe: On your next inhalation, take a deep full breath and hold it for five seconds. As you let it out, let it all the way out, and feel yourself floating down, down, deep into a very relaxing, receptive state.

Suggest: Before every meal and snack, you will take a few, calming breaths, and remember: To eat mindfully. To nourish your body. To take care of this body that carries you through the world. As you inhale fully for four seconds, and exhale slowly for eight seconds, you are remembering: before every meal and snack, you are automatically committing anew to breathing calmly. To eating mindfully. To nourishing your body, taking care of this body that carries you through the world.

Post-It: More and more, you are eating mindfully, nourishing your body, taking care. Effortlessly, you are committing to memory: Mindfully. Nourishing. Taking care. Automatically, committing anew: Mindful. Nourish. Care.

Return: Remembering to breathe, right now, and throughout the day. To take slow, refreshing breaths and return to normal alertness. Coming back to the present. Opening to this moment. Feeling refreshed, alert, present.

Reflect: Take a moment to think or write about what it would take to make your next meal or snack a little more mindful.

PRACTICE 9
Baby-Step Appreciation

If you have ever hoped to progress toward your weight-loss goal in giant steps, join the club. Then unjoin it. Unless you would really like to take one more giant step forward and two leaps back to the fridge and up a clothing size. For a refreshing change of pace, follow this script in order to cultivate the patience and perseverance you need to reach a more desirable destination: sustainable weight loss.

Focus: Settle in comfortably, set aside concerns, and take a full four seconds to inhale deeply. And give yourself eight long, slow seconds to exhale slowly. Once again, fill the lungs with breath. Then slowly, and completely, let the air all the way out.

Breathe: Finally, one more deep breath in, and this time hold it as you tighten the arm and leg muscles. Tighten, tighten, tighten, and let go . . . of the breath. Let go of the muscles. And feel yourself floating free and easy, like a raft on a summer day. So dreamy and drowsy. Floating aimlessly, easily down . . . deep into calm, comfort.

Suggest: Breathing, floating, and paying careful attention: The natural order of things is gradual change, incremental improvement. We roll over and learn to crawl before we learn to walk, run, or ride a bicycle. Different people make progress in different ways, but progress reliably moves forward in baby-steps. Imperfect, imprecise baby-steps. You are unique, and you have your own unique way of reaching your goals. [You can add some of your personal goals here.] The journey is much easier, more delightful, when you enjoy each small improvement, each and every stride forward. . . like taking a few, calming breaths before you eat, and noticing how you feel. If you feel hungry, giving yourself permission to eat. Just eat. And when you feel comfortably full, putting down your fork and turning your attention to other things.

Post-It: As you progress, slowly and surely, you are gaining confidence in yourself, coming to believe in your ability to get where you're going. To happily arrive at a healthy, sustainable weight.

Return: Slowly, surely breathing. With each new inspiration of breath, you are refreshing the relaxation that you have inspired today, and slowly shifting back to this moment, with greater awareness and renewed patience, with new eyes. You are arriving where you need to be. Right here and now.

Reflect: In what small way can you practice patience with yourself today? Will it be committing today's reflections to paper, or some other way?

PRACTICE 10
Picture of Health[7]

How do you become your vision of successful, sustainable weight loss? Embody your picture of health? The answer is the punchline to the old joke about how to get to Symphony Hall: practice, practice, practice. Do this trance over and over again.

Focus: As you make yourself comfortable, take a moment to adjust your neck and shoulder position. You can notice that a part of you is here, while the rest of you can drift off to anywhere it likes, to the middle of nowhere. A quiet inner state, where there's nothing to do. No to-dos, except breathing. Just breathing quietly, steadily, smoothly.

Breathe: And drifting away, letting yourself let go, and enter a warm, comfortable relaxation as if you were basking in the warm spring sun after a long, cold winter. That's right, imagine a welcome warmth relaxing the face muscles into a more peaceful expression. Warm relaxation flowing gently down the neck and across the shoulders. Spreading out through the chest, making it easier to breathe more quietly, steadily, smoothly. Inhaling ease, calm, peace, whatever you most need, and exhaling the rest. Rest, relaxation flowing down the lower back and through the legs. Spreading slowly but surely down the calves, down the ankles, and into the feet. The whole body softening into relaxation, calm, ease.

Suggest: Let your mind drift forward in time, to a future date, a day you can clearly see that your overeating is history. Imagine what it's like to wake up feeling good about yourself and your life. For one thing, you are no longer a slave to food. You are in charge, not food. You feel energetic, confident, comfortable in your skin and your clothes. As you look forward to the day, you fast-forward this new healthier you to a meal, any meal. Use your senses to set the scene, the table. Watch with curiosity what it's like to bring this new energy, this new respect for your body, to the table. Notice the difference, the difference in the details. Are there flowers on the table? Are you alone or with a dining companion? Could that be your favorite music playing in the background? Ideally, you would have sat down to a meal you ordered or prepared yourself from a variety of healthy, fresh foods that promise to be tasty, satisfying, and nourishing.

Focus on all that's different about you: your expression, posture, appearance, your attitude toward the meal, the eating experience from first to last forkful. Observe what it's like to chew slowly, to savor each bite, taking your time to appreciate the taste, texture, color. So different from the way you used to eat. What stands out—you no longer wonder when to stop eating. As soon as you notice you're comfortably full, satisfied, nourished, it's natural to put down your fork and turn your attention to other activities besides eating.

Post-It: Like breathing, in and out, each and every day, or practicing self-hypnosis. With every practice session, you find yourself becoming more like your healthy ideal. Believing, more and more, that the day will come, soon enough, that you like the way you look and feel. You are your picture of health.

Return: And now, drifting back to the present . . . in five slow counts. Five: Coming back . . . Four: To this room . . . Three: Slowly, surely . . . Two: Back . . . One: To this bright, new moment with appreciative eyes.

Reflect: What looks different when you try on a brighter, more hopeful viewpoint? Note the difference in your mind's eye, or even better, on notebook paper.

PRACTICE 11
Mindless Memories

Overeating is uncomfortable, you've probably noticed—not only in the moment, but for a while afterward. If only that discomfort could inform future dining decisions. To inspire healthier, more moderate portions, this trance invites you to learn from eating experiences you might prefer to forget.

Focus: Settle into comfort and a steady breathing rhythm. Breathe slowly, steadily, comfortably, and focus your mental energy on an unhealthy snack you tend to overeat. As you recall the snack's specifics—its shape, color, and texture—everyday concerns begin to fade away.

Breathe: As you continue to breathe, taking deep inhalations, long and quiet exhalations, you are inflating and deflating the tummy like a balloon. Inhaling for four seconds and think the word "deep." Exhaling for eight seconds and focus on "quiet." "Deep" for four silent seconds. "Quiet" for another eight seconds of silence.

Suggest: Once upon a time, you are casting your mind back in time . . . back to a meal or snack that you ate mindlessly. As a mindless-eating memory comes into focus, the mind recalls the scene's details—where you were, how you're sitting. Maybe you're hunching over a desk or slumping in front of the TV. Feeling what it feels like right before that first mindless morsel meets your lips. Uncomfortable, urgent, impatient. Envisioning the meal or snack, the plate or open container, the food—what it looks like, smells like, tastes like. Noticing if you bother to taste, to chew? Or if you're wolfing it down, stuffing yourself? Eating as fast as you can. Barely breathing. Shoveling it in. Your body and mind are remembering what it feels like to eat mindlessly. While you're eating . . . and then afterward. The bloat; the guilt; the self-loathing; the unhappy mix of feelings, sensations, thoughts. Your inner mind is memorizing these feelings, sensations, and thoughts to help you in the days ahead. Find time to sit . . . to breathe . . . to eat delicious, nutritious food with dignity. With respect for yourself and the food.

Post-It: You are remembering to honor yourself and the everyday activity of eating. Meal by meal, snack by snack, bite by bite.

Return: Now, as you return to deep inhalations, quiet exhalations, you are casting your mind forward to the present day, your current state of mind and body, newly aware, fully alert, happily ever now.

Reflect: Forgetting about the consequences of mindless eating is comfortably convenient, but imagine what would happen if you let yourself remember, if you would inconvenience yourself and tolerate the discomfort.

PRACTICE 12

Imaginary Triggers[8]

It's easy enough to identify the feelings, thoughts, and situations that trigger overeating; the hard part is handling triggers without overeating. Whether you are working on weight loss or maintenance, this trance makes the hard part easier. To make it even easier, start with little triggers before mentally working with bigger ones.

Focus: Invite comfort and stillness to body and mind, set aside any concerns and to-dos, and make room for calm. Inhaling calm, exhaling concerns. Inhaling calm, exhaling to-dos. As you take four silent seconds to fully inhale, think the word "calm." As you slowly exhale for eight seconds of silence, "still." "Calm" for four full seconds. "Still" for eight slow seconds of silence.

Breathe: With every breath, inviting yourself to travel deeper into relaxation. Deeper into stillness. In five slow counts, descending into the quiet stillness of inner experience. One: Focusing inward. Two: Each breath taking you. Three: Effortlessly deeper. Four: Deeper still. Five: Deep and still.

Suggest: Slim and fit. Yes, see yourself as the world will soon see you: slim and fit. Living and feeling differently about yourself because you've got a handle on your eating. For the most part, you eat healthfully, even when confronted with the feelings, thoughts, and situations that used to trigger overeating. Learn from future experience. Call to mind a triggering scene. Bring it to life with as many of your senses as you can. See it, feel it, experience what it's like to be a healthy eater in a previously unsettling scenario. What's different: your appearance, your mood, your energy? Having reached and maintained your goal of [add your own goal here], notice how you interact with others. Notice your hands, what they're doing instead of automatically reaching for food. Watch with curiosity as the scene unfolds. If at any point, a problem were to arise, pause. Breathe. Something will occur to you—a solution, a coping strategy, a healthy choice. If not instantly, in time, with practice. Stay with the scene for a few quiet moments.

Post-It: Keep in mind: the more you imagine eating healthfully in triggering or unsettling situations, the more you will be able to experience yourself as someone who eats healthfully, to feel like the you who used to overeat was someone you knew a long time ago.

Return: Now, as you deepen your breathing, refreshing the relaxation that you've inspired, you begin making your way back to your current situation, back to your immediate surroundings, back to the light of this present moment.

Reflect: Even if it's hard to imagine, try on the idea that you are learning how to effectively handle triggers and generally eat healthfully.

PART III

Mindfulness

*The Power of
Conscious Awareness*

THE CURIOUS MEDITATOR

*The curious paradox is that when I accept myself
just as I am, then I can change.*

CARL ROGERS

Before I learned to connect the dots between the age-old attention-focusing practices of mindfulness meditation and modern-day wisdom from psychology, I gave lots of lip service to eating mindfully. "Appreciate food's texture, taste, color as if you'd gone to Paris and mastered the art of French cooking," I used to suggest to clients with eating issues. Their reaction mirrored my own: "Great idea, but I'm kinda busy here, and I seem to be eating as much as always."

Fast-forward to the present, where like-minded colleagues are developing mindfulness-based treatments for the range of eating issues. In just one example, binge-eating study subjects who learned traditional breathing meditations and the latest mindful-eating techniques have been shown to eat with measurably more control and less compulsion. With a proven step-by-step approach to mindful eating, my clients began to get it. Eating, just eating while they're eating, rather than mindlessly opening mouth, inserting fork while reading the paper, watching TV, texting, or driving, they found satisfaction in less food. And they started getting better faster. Slimmer, too.

The scientific evidence was validating, but even more persuasive was client success. Watching lifetime Weight Watchers members lose weight without dieting, witnessing compulsive overeaters gain control of their eating, seeing binge eaters feel satisfied with a single slice of cake, I became more than a believer. I became a faithful practitioner, an enthusiastic proponent. (But by no means a religious fanatic. Mindfulness is not a religion.) In other words, I practiced, but did no preaching, just teaching these more effective practices.

Now, if you have tried eating mindfully and all you got for your good efforts was a bad case of the munchies, you may feel underenthused right now about giving mindful eating another go. Even if I tell you that drastic improvements in teaching techniques have decreased the likelihood of the sorry outcome of your original effort, you may be quite certain that you will never catch my contagious enthusiasm for mindfully meditating on your dinner plate. Rather than reconsider tuning in to hunger and fullness signals, you might prefer to stick your fingers in your ears and sing, "LA, LA, LA . . . "

No one can convince you to eat mindfully, and rest assured, I won't try. But I will encourage you to see for yourself after a little show and tell. I intend to *show* you the defining historical moments, key scientific research, and "aha"-inspiring meditations that spurred me on. I plan to *tell* you stories of hope resurrected, eating transformed, and figures reshaped. In the storytelling, I will be sure to translate foreign terms and concepts as needed.

TELLTALE MIND

Let's start with a lingo lesson, shall we? More than a state of mind, mindfulness is a practice that involves awareness and acceptance of the present moment. In other words, if you focus on breathing, right now, exactly as you are, you are practicing mindfulness. When your mind naturally wanders, gently bring it back to your breath. Over and over again. If you realize that you're feeling less than self-compassion-ate—dwelling on how fat you feel, beating yourself up for overeating earlier, or promising yourself to be "good" starting tomorrow—refocus on your breathing and recommit to being right here, right now, just as you are. Mindfulness, an essential component of self-compassion, is just this repeating pattern of focus, wandering, and returning to focus.

Mindful eating is bringing that same awareness and acceptance to the everyday activity of eating. Through attending to the physiological, emotional, and sensual experience of meals and snacks, mindful eaters gain access to inner wisdom, or in Jane Austen-speak, sense and sensibility: the sense to choose when, what, and how much to eat; the sensibility to learn from those choices, however virtuous.

Even a jelly donut is a worthwhile object of mindful appreciation—that is, if you permit yourself the much maligned, densely caloric treat. And stay present, without zoning out, to the full gustatory experience. The gritty sugar on fingertips, the doughy aroma that gets you salivating before your teeth sink into the soft cake or your tongue finds the cool jelly filling. The musical slurping, gurgling, and swallowing sounds more like drinking than chewing, especially for the donut dunker, who takes great pleasure in melting the gooey sweetness in her mouth with a steamy coffee chaser.

After you pass the last bite through glazed lips, mop up the remaining crumbs with sticky fingers, this ode to joy reaches its perfect, koan-like conclusion with the sound of one tongue licking.

Am I suggesting that you can slim down by savoring donuts, comforting yourself with milk and cookies, and satisfying your deepest cravings? Sounds crazy, impossible, but yes, I am. You know what's even more impossible? Facing the truth about dieting when you

Q When does mindful eating begin?

A Hard to say exactly. You could
say it starts when you put
your napkin in your lap, take
a few calming breaths, and
appreciate the meal you are
about to eat. Or you could say
mindful eating begins with
planning a nutritious, delicious
menu; or shopping for
seasonal, regional, farm-fresh
fare; or scheduling meals when
you are apt to be moderately
hungry, not ravenous. You
wouldn't be wrong if you said
it starts bright and early with a
quiet meditation or a favorite
mindfulness CD. An easier
NSQ to answer is the polar
opposite of this one:

Q When does mindful eating end?

A With your last conscious breath.

step on the scale after you've regained
what you've lost and then some. It's
a depressing image, I know, but I
bring it up to help you off the dieter's
wagon once and for all. Even if you're
not currently on it, I trust you know
the wagon I'm talking about, the one
you've fallen from more times than
you care to admit. And then there's the
surrounding territory that is wagon
country: calorically-challenged menus,
"lite" recipes, fat-free desserts. Step
away from the wagon, and a new, less
familiar view appears—the vast, relatively uncharted terrain of mindfulness.
A state that invites you to accept your
present, imperfect self, but has little
interest in the future-perfect you.

Am I really saying you can achieve
a healthy, sustainable weight while
eating to your stomach's content?
Absolutely! Am I expecting you to stake an immediate claim in this
diet-free country? No, I'm not that naïve. But I'm pretty darn confident that you will gain a greater appreciation for the entire region
when you meet the psychologist who is showing mindful eating to
be a far better thing for the range of eating issues than sliced low-
carb bread.

Jean Kristeller is the innovator of Mindfulness-Based Eating Awareness Training (MB-EAT). (Pronounce the acronym as if it were initials
and a last name: M. B. Eat.) Before Kristeller set foot on the mindful-
eating scene, it had been changing at a slow crawl. Then along came

this Indiana State University psychologist, and in two short decades, two giant steps:

1. Informed by her own research on food-intake regulation, Kristeller came up with more explicit directions for assessing when you're hungry and it's time to eat, and when you're full and it's time to move on to other activities. This is something children under age five do instinctively. Her cutting-edge techniques have virtually eliminated yesteryear's technical difficulties.[1]

2. Research is proving that mindful eating is an effective treatment for eating problems greater and smaller. As I type, Kristeller and colleagues have just finished a three-site, four-year study on weight loss, and one of those colleagues, Ruth Quillian Wolever of Duke University, has completed a sister study on weight maintenance.

   Preliminary findings suggest both studies are making good on the National Institutes of Health investment ($1.8 million for the weight-loss study alone). In the twelve-week weight-loss study, subjects trained in mindful eating lost 7 pounds on average, but a considerable number lost quite a bit more (8 to 20 pounds) and were still losing a month afterward.[2]

   In the sister study, learning mindfulness skills on top of standard behavioral strategies gave subjects no advantage in maintaining significant weight loss (about 10 percent of their body weight); across the board, subjects successfully maintained. Mindfulness training did, however, make at least two subtle but measurable differences in health and well-being—it increased "intuitive eating" (eating based on hunger and fullness signals rather than situational or emotional triggers), and decreased stress-related inflammation.[3] When Kristeller and company publish their conclusive findings, the effects will likely be felt around the world.

SWEET SUCCESS

While we eagerly await those results, there's someone else I would like you to meet. Say hello to Heidi, a binge eater and die-hard Red Sox fan who did the seemingly impossible: she stopped binging and started losing during the most unlikely season, the 2004 play-offs. You already know something about Heidi because you have read her food log in chapter 4, and because her story is every dieter's: healthy weight until she cut calories to conform to Hollywood beauty standards. The less she ate, the more she wanted to eat, until she settled into a cycle of heavy dieting and compensatory gorging.

Because this twenty-four-year-old sociology grad student looks like she could be America's next top model even when she's 20 pounds overweight, her classmates had no idea this all-American blonde shared in their all-too-common eating struggle. That after one too many 100-calorie snack packs, she too would call herself "gross" and other mean, nasty names, convinced hers was a hopeless case.

Most dieters say they'll try anything, but keep trying the same old unsuccessful strategies. What set Heidi's case apart was her willingness to try something completely different. The outcome was also atypical: she succeeded more quickly and easily than she ever dared dream.

Before I show you the secrets to Heidi's dramatic success, let me point out something nose-on-your-face obvious. Diets make dieters dumb, even smart ones like Heidi. Diets inspire one and all to override their intelligence and eat large quantities of the darnedest things. Keeping in mind all the rice cakes, fiber cereal, and other tasteless diet foods you may have consumed in your dieting lifetime, let's take a look at Heidi's first *anything*.

Scene one opens on Heidi's first mindful-eating experience. Take a look: the halogen smile illuminating the couch, that's Heidi's. The attentive eyes watching from the blue recliner, those are mine. Heidi has already taken a few moments to study the figgy-ness of a dried fig—felt its heft in her hand, looked at its deep, dusty wrinkles, inhaled its subtle, earthy scent. She's poised to sink her teeth into its chewy, gooey middle, and taste the first fig of her life.

"Hey, this is sweet," she exclaimed after swallowing the first bite.

"You sound surprised," I said.

"Well, without Splenda, bananas taste terrible!"

I couldn't imagine what she meant, but her delightful laugh suggested she had discovered something surprising and kind of embarrassing. It's amazing what you can discover when you take the time to reflect on your eating experience as Heidi did. I didn't know that she had gotten into the habit of routinely sprinkling two packets of artificial sweetener on green bananas, and another four or five on this and that over the course of the day. It's not that she had forgotten ripe fruit is naturally sweet, but she always ate the same breakfast, and with artificial sweetener, she could enjoy a morning banana, ripe or not. Plus, she confessed, she was hooked on Splenda.

Further discussion led to a greater discovery and immediate action. Overriding the subtle sweetness of real food with the super sweetness of artificial sweeteners, Heidi learned, had inadvertent consequences. Sugar substitutes, researchers believe, stimulate cravings, but do not satisfy them. These substitutes generally make it hard to track calories, assess satiety, and determine when to stop eating. As soon as Heidi realized her calorie-free sugar substitute was fueling her calorie-dense, real-sugar binges, she promptly emptied her purse of the little yellow packets tucked into its pockets and started carrying ripe fruit and other truly satisfying, real foods.

Awareness helped Heidi identify another seemingly innocuous, binge-inducing behavior. Unlike the first scene, which happened in minutes, the transformative second act unfolded over several weeks in the informal laboratory of her eating life. It was there that she discovered what researchers have found in formal lab settings: under-sleeping predictably leads to overeating and weight gain.[4]

Many dieters miss or overlook this inextricable link, but not this Red Sox fan. Tracking and reflecting on behaviors that preceded bing-ing, she could no longer ignore that chronic sleep deprivation was a personal invitation to binge. Yes, she loved night games, but if she wanted to stop binging, she would have to get more sleep, even if, God forbid, it meant reading the box scores in the morning paper. But how? Heidi couldn't imagine tucking herself in before the final pitch or sleeping in the next morning. Getting more sleep would prove more challenging than getting off Splenda.

But after nine therapy sessions and several well-timed naps, Heidi outperformed study subjects with binge-eating disorder. After a simi-lar nine-session mindfulness training group, subjects decreased their weekly binging average from four to one. They did themselves proud, but not quite as proud as my singular client. Once she caught up on sleep, Heidi hit it out of the park with zero binges per week.

SERENDIPITOUS MEETING

Now's a good time to notice where you are—what you're thinking and how you're feeling about mindful eating as a possible weight-loss route. To help you reflect on your journey thus far—how you got here, where you're going—here's a short history of mindful eating, which is, by and large, the story of paths crossing serendipitously. No doubt, you have already crossed paths with other weight-loss books, diet coaches, meditation instructors, influential someone-or-others who urged you to eat slowly, chew thoroughly, and pause between bites.

In the beginning, before the man who would become Buddha ate his first mindful meal, he was a mindless-eating Indian prince. As this timeless weight-loss fable goes, the prince got fed up with feasting, and took up fasting. Hoping to liberate himself from human suffering, he tried to kill his desire for food, but nearly killed himself in the process. Today, if he were to try to survive on one daily sesame seed and a grain of rice, he would be hospitalized for anorexia and be force-fed intravenously if he refused more nutrition. (Not the most compassionate treatment, but life-threatening eating disorders in this day and age invite drastic measures.) But back in his day, good fortune kindly intervened. A young herdsmaid happened upon the rail-thin meditator and offered him a meal of milk porridge. (I'm thinking Cream of Wheat.) In the end, the soon-to-be-enlightened one stopped starving, started eating mindfully, and discovered the central tenet of Buddhist practice known as the Fourth Noble Truth, and the American kitchen-table wisdom: everything in moderation.[5]

Many weight-loss paths crossed in the ensuing centuries, but the serendipitous crossing that brought you the mindful-eating techniques you will learn in chapter 6 happened centuries later, in the early 1980s. This historic moment also involved a young maid and a meditator, but the characters in this much later chapter each had PhDs and clinical positions at the University of Massachusetts Medical Center (UMMC): Jon Kabat-Zinn and Jean Kristeller. At this course-altering intersection, the meditator encouraged the psychologist to follow his lead and teach simple mindfulness practices to compulsive overeaters and other challenging eating cases, which she did. While the soon-to-be forefather of modern-day mindfulness helped patients with chronic medical conditions mentally scan their bodies for areas of tension and relaxation, this up-and-coming researcher instructed compulsive overeaters to take calming breaths before meals and put their forks down between bites.

But the seed of Kristeller's mindful-eating program was actually a raisin. Taking a play from Kabat-Zinn's playbook, Dr. K., as colleagues call her, introduced mindfulness with a raisin meditation, which involves eating a raisin as if it's your first. After some number of raisins, Kristeller realized that one eating meditation is a start, but it's not nearly enough to help people with real eating problems. From that realization grew the program that would be enough.[6] And the rest, as they say, is history.

Despite the fact that Kristeller once worked where I now teach—the Harvard Medical School teaching hospital, which *was* Cambridge Hospital and *is* now Cambridge Health Alliance—two decades would pass before our paths crossed at a Worcester mindfulness conference. After I savored a raisin in her experiential workshop, history did what it so often does: it repeated itself. We met, we talked, I found a better way to do what I do.

In thinking about your own journey's important intersections, keep in mind that serendipity takes many forms. For Susie Orbach, author of *Fat Is a Feminist Issue,* the groundbreaking anti-diet manifesto, serendipity was a course on compulsive overeating.[7] For anorexic turned mindful autobiographer and teacher Geneen Roth, it was Orbach's manifesto and a writing class.[8] When *French Women Don't Get Fat* author Mireille Guiliano was a chubby teen, serendipity came to the rescue in the form of an unconventional doctor with a leek soup prescription.[9] In my case, serendipity has shown up as a Zen monk with a lentil soup recipe (Ed Espe Brown), a vegetarian restaurant (the late, great Common Stock), a liberating book (Jean Antonello's *Breaking Out of Food Jail),* and a delightful colleague (mindful-eating psychotherapist Alice Rosen). For my client, the quilt artist who lost 20 pounds in ten weeks, serendipity arrived in the form of a newspaper article featuring yours truly. Like I said, serendipity is a chameleon.

But be forewarned: wrong turns can look like serendipitous crossings. There's no avoiding them, but the sooner you realize you've gone astray, the sooner you can gently return to reason and get back to a more effective and mindful eating plan—as with John Harvey Kellogg, the king of Kellogg's Corn Flakes cereal. Before dedicating himself to the morning meal, the cornerstone of every American weight-loss plan, the Corn Flakes creator got sidetracked by one Horace Fletcher, also known as The Great Masticator for his chew-yourself-slim plan. So enthralled by Fletcher's simple slimming strategy—chew each bite 100 times per minute—Kellogg wrote a snappy song to chew by. When Kellogg realized that all that mindless chewing reduced food to an unpalatable paste, he got back to eating more mindfully, and got down to the business of building a cereal empire and writing health and diet books.[10] The moral of this cautionary tale: if whatever crosses your path is unable to withstand the test of time, it ain't serendipity.

TEAM EFFORT

Kellogg, like Kabat-Zinn and Kristeller, was a visionary, as was one other forward-thinking fellow who figures heavily in the evolution of mindful eating and the overarching revolution of mindfulness in medicine. To finish this short history lesson, let me introduce Harvard cardiologist Herbert Benson. Not all that long ago, health-care providers interested in meditation and mindfulness, Benson included, were afraid to speak either "m" word. One dark night in 1967, the self-protective doctor snuck thirty-six meditators into his lab to study the effect of meditation or, as he would call it in his bestselling book, *The Relaxation Response*.[11] When his self-help book met instant international publishing success a decade later, an emboldened researcher came out of the lab to teach the world his simple, effective meditation technique for reducing high blood pressure, chronic pain, insomnia, and other common physical complaints. Benson's prescription: take two ten- to twenty-minute daily relaxation sessions, and the need to call a doctor in the morning will likely decrease.

Thanks to pioneering researchers like Benson, meditating doctors and psychotherapists have emerged from the shadows to publicly join forces with Zen monks and other lifelong meditators in the research

and development of one of the most widely studied psychological treatment approaches—mindfulness-based psychotherapy. For
an idea of just how far we have come in three decades, consider the
exponential increase in mindfulness research projects (from eighty
published studies in 1980 to twelve hundred in 2009).[12] If you're
more impressed by happy endings than statistical trends, picture this
especially historic one: at Harvard Medical School's 2009 Mindfulness and Psychotherapy Conference, Benson shared the podium with
the Dalai Lama. The eyes of a thousand health-care professionals
watched as the spirited cardiologist, thirty years into a most remarkable journey, stepped into the spotlight after His Holiness.

The payoff of all this scientific team effort is a choice of proven treatments to decrease depression, anxiety, stress, and pain (the physical
sensation and the emotional distress); increase relaxation, immunity,
and mental acuity; and generally improve health and well-being. The
choice of treatment extends to eating issues. In addition to Kristeller's
MB-EAT, there are more than a half dozen programs with matching acronyms: Dialectical Behavior Therapy (DBT), Acceptance
and Commitment Therapy (ACT), Mindfulness-Based Cognitive
Therapy (MBCT), Appetite Awareness Training (AAT), and Enhanc-
ing Mindfulness for the Prevention of Weight Regain (EMPOWER).
I have yet to make an acronym for my Integrative Mindful-Eating
Therapy. (I-MET doesn't quite do it for me.)

Forget about keeping the acronyms straight, and remember these
exciting findings: mindful-eating training has been shown to help veteran dieters eat with markedly more control, and has enabled binge
eaters to binge significantly less (both the number of binges per week
and the amount of food per binge). Mindful eaters generally feel less
depressed and anxious, and face a decreased risk of diabetes and other
weight-related health problems. They even metabolize food better
than their mindless friends, evidenced in reduced insulin sensitivity.[13]

Enquiring minds, I know, are most interested to know if mindful eating facilitates weight loss. The first large-scale study of a targeted mindfulness treatment for obese and overweight individuals will soon be published, but less rigorous studies have already shown what my clients have demonstrated: waist watchers who faithfully practice meditation and mindful eating do lose weight. It's worth repeating: if you make mindfulness practice a part of your routine, you will likely lose weight without dieting. The advance word from three such studies is encouraging.

1. The nineteen subjects who learned mindful-eating and distress-tolerance skills in an ACT weight-loss study lost about 7 percent of their body weight in twelve weeks. And over the next six months, they lost another 3 percent, for a total of 10 percent.[14]
2. A survey of four thousand-plus Japanese adults revealed that eating mindlessly—eating too quickly to recognize moderate fullness—is associated with being overweight. Compared to self-described mindful-eating subjects, mindless eaters registered higher body weights and scores on the body mass index, the standardized body-fat measure.[15]
3. The study that inspires the biggest WOW! is one of the smallest, a case study of a 315-pound man who, as a result of individual mindful-eating therapy, lost and maintained 144 pounds.[16]

Why would meditating on a raisin, an enchilada, or a Twinkie for that matter, help you eat with more restraint and weigh less? Because eating mindfully heightens your awareness of hunger and fullness cues, helps you tolerate the distressing feelings, thoughts, and circumstances that inspire overeating, or, at the very least, makes it possible to delay the urge to overeat long enough to find a healthier way of coping.

Mindfulness training works on an even deeper level. According to a growing body of research, you are able to think, feel, and behave differently because mindfulness practices actually rewire the brain and reprogram the body. If after two months of regular practice, you were to wear a snug wig of electrodes to record brain activity, you could expect the electroencephalograph (EEG) to reveal enhanced electrical activity in areas of the brain associated with positive emotions. If you were to also volunteer for a blood test, the lab tech would likely find an elevated level of antibodies, evidence of enhanced immunity. If while you were meditating you happened to be hooked up to biofeedback equipment, you would notice a healthier heart rate—more specifically, an increase in heart-rate variability, a measure of nervous system functioning. But paradoxically, you could detect a slightly faster breathing rhythm. Learning to pay careful attention tends to increase the breathing rate initially and ever so slightly, but in time, reliably and significantly decreases it. And if you continued a meditation practice into your twilight years and were to slide into an MRI machine for a brain scan, the X-ray tech would see a younger-looking brain, thicker in attention-related areas that naturally thin with age.[17]

When you add up all the benefits, it's hard to imagine who wouldn't be interested in mindful eating. Who in their right mind wouldn't be more than a little curious about the prospect of losing weight without dieting? Who wouldn't enjoy living more healthfully and happily ever after?

EMPOWERING TREATMENT

Mindfulness training programs vary in every possible way—content, clientele, and length. Mindfulness programs for eating issues range from one to twenty-three sessions, and take place in therapist-led groups, although some, like mine, serve up lessons to individual clients. All mindfulness trainings, including mindful-eating programs, share the same ambitious goal: awareness without judgment and with acceptance, if not a touch of loving-kindness. Most trainings also share one essential practice: silent meditation.

When meditation is a formal part of the lesson plan, early instruction includes sitting or lying with a relaxed focus on the breath, and when the attention naturally wanders, refocusing on the breath over and over again. To help new meditators extend this focused attention to daily life, they are typically encouraged to incorporate walking meditation or yoga into their lives. From day one, there's homework, usually some amount of daily meditation, ranging from three to sixty minutes, but averaging twenty to thirty minutes a day. It's helpful to think of this mental training like physical workouts. Just as you can play a sport, albeit poorly, without building muscle strength, you can eat more mindfully without developing mental strength. But if you really want to gain success, you need to train. Or to rephrase the old workout motto: no training, little or no attaining.

Eating mindfully is far from a foreign concept. We learn some of the essential practices early and informally through some combination of family tradition, proper etiquette, and religious ritual. As soon as we leave the high chair for the dining room table, we are encouraged to practice mindfulness—sit down, maybe say grace, place napkin in lap, fork in hand.

When it's taught more formally as part of mindful-eating training, lessons often take the form of guided meditations. A guided meditation on hunger awareness, for example, invites trainees to focus on personal hunger cues, noticing if they're hungry, approximately how hungry, and how they know how hungry they are.[18] Awareness makes it possible to notice how hunger asks, then demands attention through bodily sensations, thoughts, and feelings. If you were a fly on the wall after a group hunger-awareness meditation, you would hear the many different ways hunger speaks to different people. Palpable sensations are easiest to perceive. Some mindful eaters are able to sense the vague emptiness in the abdomen of mild hunger, while many remain clueless until hunger pangs clearly signal they're ravenous. Hunger, you would also learn, communicates through thoughts and feelings. Mild hunger might whisper to you in fleeting food-focused thoughts or passing restless feelings; extreme hunger is more apt to shout for attention with obsessive planning and explosive irritability.

Detecting fullness is a no-brainer twenty minutes after eating, but given how many calories we can all mindlessly consume in fewer than five, it pays to pay attention early. A guided meditation on stomach fullness teaches mindful eaters a new respect for the body part that gets next to none from dieters: the heart of the digestive system. This particular meditation trains attention on the subtle and not-so-subtle fullness signals as they arise in the abdomen. (For a Personal Slimming Lesson on fullness cues, don't miss the one titled, "Am I Full Yet?")

PERSONAL SLIMMING LESSON

Am I Full Yet?

You are hardwired to recognize fullness when blood sugar rises twenty minutes after a meal. But you've probably noticed that you can eat a lot in twenty minutes, especially when you're stressed or starving. If only there were a warning system to alert you earlier, spare you the distress of snugger pants, harsher self-criticisms. There is, but most waist watchers have never learned how to use it.

Wanna learn? Try this at the next meal or snack: Start by tuning in to the clearest satiety signals from the abdomen and taste buds. From bite one, stay alert to the building sensation of your tummy filling up, waistband tightening, taste intensity diminishing. Next do a head-to-toe scan for the subtler fullness cues: muscles relaxing, food looking and smelling less appetizing, attention shifting from eating to other activities, legs and feet readying to move along. Keep checking for your personal signals; you may notice other cues.

As you continue eating, check back for the full range of fullness cues, and intermittently ask yourself: "Am I full yet?" When all or most signs point to "yes," when you're pretty sure you're comfortably full, put down your fork and move away from the table. Etiquette permitting, of course.

Another meditation that helps mindful eaters decide when to stop eating focuses on taste-specific satiety, the technical term for the taste buds' decreasing ability to find pleasure in a particular food's flavor. This law of diminishing taste-bud sensation is the reason why you eventually get bored with chicken Caesar salad, but can still delight in a switch to chocolate ice cream. People keep eating partly to regain that initial burst of flavor, even though it isn't going to happen. Meditating on how quickly your taste buds tire of the same taste doesn't prevent you from overeating, but it does make it easier to put down your parfait spoon before you polish off the whole pint.

Like yesteryear's skiing lessons on graduated skis, some programs take an incremental approach, starting with meditations on neutral foods (raisins, cheese and crackers) and working up to treats that many dieters are afraid to keep in the cupboard (chips, cookies, chocolate cake). Rather than giving participants carte blanche to mindfully eat whatever they want, these bite-sized lessons help them face fears and build confidence surely, but not necessarily slowly. The fact that graduates have gone on to take all-inclusive cruises without gorging is testimony to the success of this baby-stepping approach.

Other programs distinguish themselves in other ways. One concentrates on fat-related fears and other unsettling thoughts that trigger overeating; another focuses on managing the emotions that fuel emotional overeating; a third aims to develop coping behaviors besides eating that embody personal values and overarching goals. Lessons in self-compassion, inner wisdom, and forgiveness of oneself and one's body are often an implicit, and sometimes explicit, part of the lesson plan.

None of the treatments endorse a specific diet or food plan, though at least one offers diet and exercise guidelines. The rationale for this diet-free approach to eating issues: when you stop trying to control your intake—stop counting carbs, calories, and points—you start eating with a greater sense of control. Clients who have dieted for decades aren't necessarily eager or interested in ditching their diets for this radical, paradoxical, un-American weight-loss approach. And they don't have to. In fact, some dedicated dieters find mindful eating helps them stick more closely to their food plan. Others derive an enormous benefit from training their awareness on the experience of dieting—noticing how puny portions affect their hunger; if diet foods please their palate; what it's like to do the math and realize they have met their daily caloric allotment long before dinner. If and when it becomes clear that undereating is fueling their overeating, dieters are often more interested in taking a break from dieting and seeing what happens when they focus exclusively on mindful eating as the slimming plan.

New clients in search of a quick fix aren't particularly interested in the long-term investment of mindful eating. Given the choice between hypnosis and eating mindfully, they choose the magic cure that they perceive hypnosis to be over the hard work they imagine mindfulness involves. I'm happy to give them what they want, plus a little more. I make mindful-eating lessons more palatable by delivering them as hypnotic suggestions: "You'll find yourself eating more slowly," I suggest, "and naturally losing weight." It's a little sneaky, I admit, but in most cases the results are magical. Clients who do well on my Hypnotic-Responsiveness Quiz and prove to be hypnotically responsive are delighted to discover themselves automatically eating more slowly—and naturally losing weight.

It makes sense that good hypnotic subjects make talented mindful eaters. Research has shown that the ability to focus or get mentally absorbed predicts both superior hypnotic talent and deeper meditative experience.[19] If you have talent for getting lost in thought or daydreams, and you skipped the hypnosis section, you might want to reconsider the power of positive suggestion.

FINDING THINSPIRATION

Eat Seasonal, Regional

Some dieters are so busy "being good," trying to satisfy themselves with supermarket grapefruits and iceberg lettuce, they forget to notice the local markets overflowing with local strawberries and corn. These are the same gals who, rather than bicycling outdoors on the most glorious June day, try to force themselves into the dank gym to lift weights. Sound like anyone you know?

If you've been wondering *why* it's impossible to stick to a slimming plan or *if* you can't lose weight because of a metabolic malfunction, a chemical imbalance, or something worse, try asking yourself a most radical question: "What would please my palate?" Or as my mindful colleague Alice Rosen likes to ask: "What are you humming for?" On long summer days and warm lazy evenings, we typically "hum" for lighter, simpler meals alfresco—picnics at the beach or hot off the backyard grill. We have emerged from the dark of winter hibernation into longer, lighter days craving lower-fat, lower-calorie entrees featuring fresh produce and garden herbs. A more active lifestyle, too. Come fall, we retreat to the kitchen for comfort food—hot cereal, hearty stews and soups. And turn to winter sports or head back to the gym.

That's just the way it is. Breakfasting on grapefruit year-round is a good formula for boredom and weight gain. Delighting in the seasonal bounty, planning menus around farm-fresh regional fare, now that's a delightful recipe for Thinspiration and sustainable weight loss.

GOOD CANDIDATE

What characterizes a good candidate for mindfulness training? First and foremost, the human condition. Membership in the human race comes with lifetimes of suffering, as the Buddhist teachings explain, and mindfulness reliably relieves, if not stops, the suffering. Better candidates for mindful-eating training are not only all too aware of suffering, but a major source of their suffering has become the human need for food. Candidates don't struggle with the same eating problems, but they all share a genuine interest in feeding themselves with less compulsion and more ease. Good candidates are people with weight-related health problems (high blood pressure, joint problems, diabetes, heart disease), everyday eating disturbances (yo-yo dieting, emotional eating, compulsive overeating), or diagnosable eating disorders (bulimia, binge-eating disorder, and bulimarexia—alternating cycles of bulimia and anorexia). Even dieters who have succeeded in reaching a healthy weight but feel they have failed to meet societal beauty standards have something to gain.

Like May, a forty-two-year-old professor who was well acquainted with feeling ravenous, but a stranger to mild and moderate hunger. Before a short course of mindful-eating therapy, this extreme dieter, who once trained for a marathon on 600 calories a day, used to chastise herself for eating muffins midmorning. "I had no idea I was hungry," May exclaimed after learning to recognize lesser degrees of hunger. Getting to know her hunger didn't happen overnight, but proved an essential early step to preventing that impulsive, no-foods-barred state she described as "hide the dogs and small children." Once she could recognize the physiological signals of hunger, the next important step was allowing herself to heed the signals and feed herself over the course of the day. Developing a healthy respect for hunger and its alter ego, fullness, took time, but it also took off 32 pounds in thirty-two weeks.

People with eating disorders, as well as those with eating problems that fall short of diagnosable disorders, have found mindful eating invaluable. Whether they binge many times a day or just once a year, people who binge are pained by their inability to stop eating, not by starting to eat too often. To stop binging, they need to learn what May learned—to recognize and respond to fullness cues. Mindful eating teaches binge eaters how to do just that. The same judgment-free awareness could be literally lifesaving for anorexics, whose recovery depends on their ability to start and finish a meal despite an acute sensitivity and negative reaction to feeling full. Existing programs cater to overeaters, not undereaters. Currently, if you're interested in mindful eating and suffer from anorexia or another eating problem involving calorie restriction, individual psychotherapy is your best and only training option.

Mindful eating has much to offer patients of bariatric surgery (gastric bypass, lap-band, and so forth). To increase the surgery's short- and long-term effectiveness, more hospitals are offering lessons in mindfulness as part of patient education. The surgery itself, patients say, heightens awareness of stomach satiety, but that awareness isn't enough to inhibit unhealthy eating habits or binge eating, which plagues a significant number of surgery candidates and can lead to post-surgical failures. The extent to which surgery impacts post-surgical patients' ability to recognize fullness is unclear, but mindfulness can clearly help them savor the prescribed smaller portions and recognize feelings and thoughts that have fueled emotional overeating.[20]

Take it from Edie, a fifty-seven-year-old travel agent who recently underwent laparoscopic gastric bypass. "I lost 70 pounds in four months," said Edie, twirling to show off her girlish figure and stretchy black Eileen Fisher dress. "But I still listen to mindful-eating CDs. They help me eat slowly." Mindful-eating lessons from individual psychotherapy also helped Edie discover that she didn't have to bore her palate with diet chocolate shakes and other processed food products. If she enjoyed a steady diet of nutritious, delicious real food, she could count on her taste buds to let her know when the gustatory thrill was gone, and it was time to move on to life's other pleasures, like knitting and watching *American Idol*.

Mindful eating also holds promise for unsuccessful dieters with attention deficit disorder (ADD) and its cousin ADHD (*h* for hyperactivity.) Obese people are three to five times more likely to be diagnosed with attention issues, but most are unaware that, without proper treatment, these diagnoses are one of the main reasons it's so darned hard to lose weight. The ADD brain is quicker to lose focus, but slower to metabolize sugar. This makes it hard to consistently stick to a diet and easy to overdose on sweets before the perception of satiety sets in. Overwhelmed by the food shopping, menu planning, and meal scheduling that slimming plans require, dieters with ADD seek comfort in what their more attentive friends would consider sickly sweet treats (coffee with umpteen sugars, full-sugar soda by the gallon).[21] Hard to believe, but to their taste buds, supersweet usually tastes just right.

With therapy, I'm happy to report, lonely weight battles become winnable wars. In fact, weight loss is an unintended benefit of ADD treatment, usually some mix of medication, psychotherapy, and increasingly meditation. Meditation, as you've been learning, increases activity in brain regions used for paying attention. The longer you train with meditation, the more you stand to gain. But a little practice can go a long way. By meditating just twenty minutes for five consecutive days, Chinese college students who practiced a variation of mindfulness meditation outperformed their relaxation-technique-practicing classmates on tests of attention.[22] (It's worth noting: meditation is not simply relaxation, but relaxation is the natural result of regular meditation.)

DIFFERENT DRUMMER

Time is short, or at least it seems so, and mindful eating takes time. In our fast-food nation, it has become a real challenge to squeeze in three square meals a day. If and when the family finally sits down for dinner, place settings are often set beside laptops and BlackBerries. The only family members who insist on eating meals on any consistent schedule are Fido and Fluffy. Even schoolchildren have little time for lunch. One client's daughter was encouraged by her school to take an advanced placement class in lieu of lunch. When this honors student was diagnosed with an eating disorder, the mom had to get special permission for her daughter to snack in the nurse's office.

Waist watchers may be short on time, but not cash. Last I checked, the dieting industry was collecting $35–40 billion a year. As if dieters weren't naturally fixated enough on quick fixes, the makers of diet products and slimming programs promise that their plan makes it possible to lose 10 pounds in the blink of a false eyelash. You won't hear empty promises from mindful-eating proponents, but you will hear the occasional celebrity endorsement from the likes of chef Alice Waters, mother of the Slow Food Movement. That's the global effort to improve quality of life by improving quality of food. And comedienne Margaret Cho, who has spoken publicly about casting off diets and the eating disorders they inspire, and embracing a "whatever" diet. Mindfully eating whatever—French fries, pizza—a more accepting, less self-critical Cho dropped 40 pounds. "You get to the understanding that not everybody's a size 2," Cho confided to a *People* magazine reporter. "Sometimes you're a size 12—and you're still beautiful."[23]

Once Kristeller, the diligent researcher, meets the press to discuss her latest weight-loss study findings, more waist watchers may give mindful eating a try. But because doing anything mindfully means marching to the beat of a different, unpopular drummer, don't expect your friends to fall in line. And don't expect mindful eating to catch on like the South Beach Diet. Only you can choose to eat more mindfully. Only you can decide to travel the route of mindful weight loss, to arrive at a healthy, sustainable weight eating your favorite foods in moderation, with more pleasure and less guilt than diets allow. Only you can give up on indigestion, obesity, and the other unhappy, not so healthy, or uncompassionate consequences of overeating by looking for satisfaction in the quality, rather than the quantity, of food. Dieting often overlooks the satisfactions of eating: letting yourself enjoy good food in good company; allowing yourself to eat to your stomach's content; giving yourself permission to eat for relaxation or reward. Without satisfaction, dieters are doomed to regain whatever

they lose. But by allowing for satisfaction and choosing to pay attention to your body's signals, it's possible to have some cake, eat it too,
and lose weight.

PARADOXICAL MISSION

There is one catch to mindful eating that can sound like a Catch-
22: You get where you're going by staying in the here and now. You
achieve lasting weight loss by focusing on the present, not the future
and how great you'll feel when:

- you stop overeating and start working out
- you invest in a spa vacation and divest yourself of 10 pounds
- you find smaller jeans and true love

It's not that you forget about the future altogether. You can't, and if
you try, you'll succeed at thinking of nothing but the future. Success
doesn't require that degree of nearsightedness. In fact, it makes good
sense to begin with a dual focus on present and future. To set future
goals based on present reality, and then set them aside. Why? Because
now is the only time you can effect change, the only moment you can
accomplish your mission. Sure, it's natural to envision a better tomorrow, but if you focus on it, you abandon your mission for a dream. In
reality, you can never claim success as fast as your crash-dieting sister, your tummy-tucking cousin, your stomach-stapling neighbor, or
your faster-metabolizing younger self. But in making such unfavor-
able comparisons, you *can* call yourself all kinds of mean, nasty names.
You can undermine your success and reach the opposite ambition: eat
mindlessly instead of mindfully. Gain weight instead of losing weight.

Your mission, if you choose to accept it, is to eat mindfully without
striving for any particular outcome. Your challenge flies in the face
of dieting tradition—to go on a strict diet before you take vacations,

attend weddings, or make a grand appearance at other important events. You must accept yourself at your current weight. Just as you are. It might take time to work up to it. Getting into the accepting spirit of mindful eating is an evolving process.

Take it from Dina, a recovering bulimic who never imagined doing what many American women consider unimaginable—she went to her twenty-fifth high-school reunion without first going on a diet. "I used to be enslaved to the diet mentality," said Dina, triumphant in her new lack of interest in old calorie-counting ways. "Not now!" Now, two-plus decades into her recovery from bulimia, there's no healthier way for this forty-five-year-old ski instructor to go than diet-free. There's no better way to maintain her 65-pound weight loss than eating mindfully, exercising regularly, and relaxing more than occasionally. That, and remembering it's OK to love thy neighbor *and* thyself. Contrary to her religious upbringing, Dina's learned from reliable sources, including Sharon Salzberg's bestselling *Lovingkindness,* that taking care of yourself isn't prideful; it's self-compassionate. "I'm wowed by the power of self-compassion," she adds. Definitely take it from Dina: mindful eating is an evolving process, and an incredibly liberating one.

It's a useful exercise to set long-term goals as you did in the previous chapter, but once set, set them aside. Set aside future fantasies and past regrets too. Focus on the present task of living life moment by moment, meal by meal. Weight loss happens naturally when you view eating as an opportunity to expand your attention beyond the food on your plate, beyond the external dining experience, to encompass the internal terrain of mind and body. It's amazing what you will find when you stop multitasking and just eat. Simply eat. Eating becomes

THINK SELF-KIND THOUGHTS

Your Inner Critic:

I hate my _____ (*your least favorite body part*). If money could buy me anything, that'd be one of the first things I would buy.

Your Compassionate Response:

_____

_____

_____

_____

nothing less than a chance to discover who you are, how you feel, what you need. Eating becomes a standing invitation to embrace life.

No one makes this point better than Thich Nhat Hanh, the venerable Vietnamese monk. The following quote from his meditation on an orange is worth savoring: "When you are truly here, contemplating the orange, breathing and smiling, the orange becomes a miracle. It is enough to bring you a lot of happiness. You peel the orange, smell it, take a section, and put it in your mouth mindfully, fully aware of the juice on your tongue. This is eating an orange in mindfulness. It makes the miracle of life possible. It makes joy possible."[24]

MINDFUL-EATING SUGGESTIONS FOR SAVORING EACH BITE

The irony of your present eating habits is that while you fear missing a meal, you aren't fully aware of the meals you do eat.

DAN MILLMAN

In theory, mindful eating sounds easy. Eat when you're hungry, stop when you're full, and you'll naturally reach your desired weight...without dieting. In other words, pay attention—gentle, nonjudgmental attention—to the everyday act that is eating. In practice, mindful weight-loss programs are more challenging than most diets because they ask waist watchers to notice things they might like to ignore—the sensation of hunger and fullness for starters—and they are far more challenging than diet plans that provide individual meals and snacks in stocking-stuffer-sized packages.

Yup, mindful eating is easier said than done, but for so many reasons, it's worth doing. If you have yet to see reason enough, well, you could always review chapter 5. But you don't need to be completely sold on mindful eating to explore this less familiar territory. In fact, whatever your current view of weight loss, there's something to be said for just trying on a more mindful viewpoint. Seeing what you can see, finding what you can find.

In this sixth chapter, you will find answers to FAQs (Frequently Asked Questions), also known as NSQs (No Stupid Questions), and much more. To start, there's a quiz. It will help you assess how mind-fully you currently live, breathe, and eat. Once you begin to integrate mindfulness practices into your life, you will take it again later to see how far you've come. In between, you will learn a total of eight mind-ful breathing and eating practices. These are the very same practices that have helped my clients realize their weight-loss goals, and in the process achieve other life dreams. To keep your dreams from turning into nightmares, I will teach you how to incrementally face the foods you tend to overeat. Food by food, bite by bite, breath by breath.

If you opened directly to this chapter hoping to find a diet, you can stop looking. You won't find menu plans or food lists in this or any other chapter. Everything you need for mindful weight loss is right here—a quiz, and the suggested practices. Or as I like to call them, the suggestions. There's just one prerequisite: an open mind.

The quiz you are about to take is based on two scientific measures: the Mindful Eating Questionnaire and the Philadelphia Mindfulness Scale.[1] Mine may be less scientific, but it's more accessible. And you don't need a PhD to score it. More like your bathroom scale than the one at the doctor's office, what my quiz lacks in accuracy it makes up for in convenience and privacy. Strive to answer each question as honestly as you can. If you find yourself craving a high score more than a fair assessment, pause. Deepen your inhalation, lengthen your exhalation. This craving will pass. They always do.

QUIZ 3
Jean's Mindful-Eating Quiz

Take this quiz and find out how mindful you are. After cultivating mindful awareness for at least a week (via the practices in this chapter), take the quiz again. When you compare your scores, you'll discover what a measurable difference mindfulness makes to your ability to focus and follow your healthiest instincts. Consider how often the twenty-one statements below describe you, just you, in the past week. Next to each statement, note one of the following: never/rarely (n/r), sometimes (s), often (o), almost always/always (u/a).

_____   1. Even if I'm enjoying a favorite food, I stop eating when I'm comfortably full.

_____   2. When confronted with a supersized snack, I tend to overeat.

_____   3. I don't care if the large portion is a bargain, I order according to hunger, not price.

_____   4. Candy, birthday cake, you name it, if it's there I'll eat it.

_____   5. Before picking up my fork, I pause to appreciate the food on my plate.

_____   6. I eat so quickly, I barely taste what I'm eating.

_____   7. I notice if the chef has a heavy hand with the salt shaker.

_____   8. If I start eating something, I'll finish it even if it's not all that tasty.

_____   9. Even when movie theater popcorn looks or smells tempting, I'll only buy a bag when I'm truly hungry and specifically wanting a salty, crunchy snack.

_____   10. If it's mealtime, I'm eating a meal even if I'm not the least bit hungry.

_____   11. I notice the effect of food on my mood.

_____   12. I wish I had better control of a lot of things, especially my appetite.

_____   13. If I choose to comfort myself with food, it's a conscious, thoughtful choice.

_____   14. As soon as my least favorite feeling rears its ugly head, I stuff it down with food.

_____   15. When my attention naturally wanders from my dinner plate, I bring it back and refocus on the dining experience.

_____ 16. When I eat, I find at least one other thing to do:
             reading, watching TV, texting.

_____ 17. Come mealtime, I set aside what I'm doing and
             focus on the meal.

_____ 18. If I notice I'm hungry, I look for a distraction to
             keep me from eating.

_____ 19. I try to eat a nutritious diet, but forbid myself nothing.

_____ 20. If I've overeaten, I try to avoid reflecting on the
             whole experience, especially the uncomfortable feelings
             and sensations.

_____ 21. I generally accept my body, imperfections and all.

Scoring Sheet

For the odd-numbered statements, give yourself 1 point for each
"never/rarely"; 2 for "sometimes"; 3 for "often"; 4 for "almost always/
always." For each even-numbered statement, give yourself 1 for "almost
always/always"; 2 for "often"; 3 for "sometimes"; 4 for "never/rarely."

Record your total on the line below:

Total Score: _____   Date: _____ / _____ / _____

Your Score and What to Make of It

When it comes to mindfulness, 21–42 means you can only go up from
here; 43–72, you are moderately mindful in a mindless society, but
there's room for improvement; 73–84, you are wise beyond your dieting peers. More aware and self-accepting, too. Bravo!

Take this test again after a week or two of mindfulness practice. If
you initially scored low, your progress will be most remarkable. If
you're already pretty mindful, know that even a slight increase will
help you improve your eating habits and, yes, lose weight. And if you

would like to earn the big health and well-being dividends, invest (or reinvest) in regular mindfulness practice.

MINDFUL-EATING SUGGESTIONS

There are so many different ways to cultivate mindfulness. To make your choice much simpler, this section gives you two types of practices in two subsections: The Breathing Practices and The Eating Practices. Breathing comes before eating because mindful breathing helps you attend to whatever you are thinking, feeling, and doing, including eating. The six eating practices focus more specifically on food, giving you insight into what you are eating (or about to eat) and what's potentially eating you.

If you've tried any of the previous practices, you are pretty well-prepared for this chapter's breathing practices. The eating meditations, however, take a little extra preparation. If these practices are the first you are trying, the best way to get ready is to review "How to Read This Book." Second best: read this brief recap of general practice preparations.

Ready: Mindfulness practice takes time, about fifteen to twenty minutes a day. You will benefit most from one continuous session, but if you're a new meditator or crazy busy, there's a lot to be said for several shorter sessions. If short and sweet sounds like your best bet, you'll want to Float (that's the name of the second breathing practice) at least once, if not several times, over the course of the day. For the biggest daily benefit, the better bet is Breathe, the longer breathing practice. Feel free to lengthen either practice by adding stretches of silence here and there.

THINK SELF-KIND THOUGHTS

Your Inner Critic:

People say 'Love me, love my imperfections,' but I don't want to love my imperfections. They're unlovable, as am I.

Your Compassionate Response:

_____

_____

_____

_____

All the mindful-eating meditations are beneficial, but they're especially beneficial if you take a full fifteen to twenty minutes to practice by mindfully setting the table, serving the food, sitting down, breathing, and eating. What you want to avoid doing, at least intentionally, is making a regular practice of the Mindless-Eating Meditation. Anytime is the right time to practice mindful breathing, but the best time to develop your mindful-eating skills is when you're more than a little hungry, but not ravenous.

Set: Practicing mindfulness also takes space, one that's safe, quiet, and comfortable. If you can find comfort on a meditation cushion, go ahead and make yourself comfortable. Otherwise, do the breathing meditations sitting or lying down wherever you like. The eating meditations are best done sitting, preferably near a table or another flat surface. With both types of practice, you might enhance the scene's serenity with candlelight or soothing background music. Also, do what you can to minimize distractions—close the door, dim the lights, and turn off your cell phone. But once you've started a practice, keep at it even if distractions pop up. Acknowledge and accept inevitable distractions as invitations to refocus on the object of your meditation.

Practice: Try all the practices at least once, and repeat the most helpful ones as long as you find them helpful. If you're serious about making mindfulness a sustainable weight-loss strategy, seriously consider making a daily routine of Breathe, the longer breathing practice, and the All-Purpose Eating Meditation, the last eating meditation.

Generally you should try to stick to the script the first time through a practice. But instead of simply reading it as you would a magazine article, mindfully focus on the words and any images that are suggested. Once you've got the gist of a practice, consider closing your eyes and mentally guiding yourself script-free.

Because multitasking cultivates mindlessness, it makes good mindful sense to make reading and eating separate activities. Before you try an eating meditation, read the instructions until you can envision the practice without the script, then eat as instructed. Another mindful way to go: read a bit, take a bite, read another bit, take another bite. The usual options remain good options: enlist a willing reader, record and replay your own reading voice, or listen to *The Self-Compassion Diet* audio. After the reading, when you're into eating, heighten the experience by closing your eyes for a few bites. When you've finished eating, but before you rush to the next activity, stay put and reflect on your experience.

THE BREATHING PRACTICES

Breathing is the simplest, handiest tool for cultivating mindfulness—and therefore mindful eating. Volumes have been written about why the automatic activity of breathing loosens the iron grip of obesity and other eating problems, but you will find reason enough to make a practice of mindful breathing in this short explanation:

When you "Breathe, just breathe," as songwriter Anna Nalick suggests, your body relaxes, your mind awakens. Create a regular time and space to "just breathe." It's a self-compassionate act. It gives you perspective on eating patterns that escape everyday awareness, and a chance to change those patterns. When the mid-afternoon munchies strike, for example, rather than bolting for the vending machine, a mindful-breathing practice makes it possible to sit still long enough to assess if your hunger is emotional or physical, and how best to satisfy it. Instead of making do with the instant gratification of a candy bar or a bag of chips, you have a real chance of making lasting change when you take the time to breathe. Just breathing restores what dieting threatens to destroy—the vital connection between mind and body.

Dress for Success

I don't know how many new clients tell me they won't buy new clothes until they lose weight, but it's the overwhelming majority. These folks insist on making do with old, ill-fitting clothes until they drop a size or two. Perhaps you're one of those people. Experience has taught me that postponing clothes shopping contributes more to weight gain than loss. That those who refuse to trade in their threadbare fashions more often than not go up a size, not down, when they next shop.

Far more likely to succeed are those who are willing to dress for success and comfort before, not after, they reach their desired weight. Something about wearing attractive, comfortable clothes inspires waist watchers to eat more healthfully, and generally take better care of themselves. Surely you don't have to buy a new wardrobe to find Thinspiration, but it really does help to step out of those baggy sweatpants and into more form-fitting fashions. Not only does wearing something comfortably form-fitting buoy your mood, it heightens awareness of stomach fullness. It's win-win, really.

PRACTICE 13

Breathe—The Longer Practice

Mindful eating is like building a house: it pays to lay a solid foundation. Think of this fifteen- to twenty-minute breathing practice as your foundation. While it's possible to eat mindfully without meditating on the breath, it becomes far easier with a daily practice like this one.

Settle into a comfortable, dignified posture—spine straight, shoulders relaxed, arms and hands at your sides or in your lap. Soften your facial expression, and settle your attention on the breath. Allow the breath to ease into a quiet, natural rhythm. Without forcing any big inhalations or loud exhalations, the breath naturally deepens and lengthens. Inhale fully for four silent seconds, exhale slowly and completely for eight seconds of silence.

Intentionally focus on one vital aspect of your breathing. You might choose to focus on the nostrils, noticing how the air is cooler on the inhalation, warmer on the exhalation. You might find it easier to focus on the tummy, attending to the movements of your belly as air flows in and out of your body. If sound is more compelling than sensation, you might prefer to direct your attention to the ears, listening to the wavelike whispers of inhalations and exhalations. Feel free to experiment with several focal points before anchoring your attention on one.

When you notice your attention naturally wander from your focal point, become aware of where it went and gently bring it back to the breath. With the kindness and patience you would offer a puppy learning to "stay," bring your attention back to the breath over and over again. In the beginning, when you tell a puppy to stay, it might sit for a moment before it gets up and walks away. You wouldn't scold it. You would pick it up, put it back, and remind it to stay—until it can stay longer and longer all by itself. Same with the mind. When the mind naturally wanders, bring it back to the breath over and over again—until it can stay longer and longer. Without judging if you're doing it right. Without worrying if there's something wrong with you. Without comparing yourself to those who seem to have an easier time of it. If your mind has more in common with a crabby two-year-old than an adorable puppy, shower it with affection. And keep on doing what you're doing: bring your focus back to the breath. Again, and again, and again.

When you can, notice what's on your mind. Observe any and all thoughts without mentally running away with them or letting them keep you from gently refocusing on the breath. Even your meanest, most critical thoughts deserve your full attention. Where is your mind right now? Is it here? Or mired in the past, thinking about what you shouldn't have eaten? Or planning for the future? Vowing to be "good" starting tomorrow or Monday or when you get back from vacation? Observe your mind, notice its contents, return to the breath.

Similarly, if a bodily sensation enters your awareness, note the sensation. Whether it's pleasant, unpleasant, or neutral, notice what it is without mentally turning toward or away from it. Whatever you notice—a tense muscle, an itch, a craving—observe the sensation without forcing or willing it away. Notice what happens when you stop resisting a persistent sensation and stop insisting it be different right now. When you just let it be.

Feelings have a way of ebbing and flowing, too. When feelings arise, pay careful attention to what's really happening. Notice the qualities that make these feelings unique and distinctive. Notice what makes you more or less curious about a certain emotion. What makes it easier or more difficult to sit with a particular feeling? Whatever the feeling, do your best to acknowledge it, accept it, and then refocus on the breath.

Like feelings, thoughts, and sensations, sounds may divert your attention and derail your focus. If you observe audible or inaudible distractions, remember that puppy. With as much loving-kindness and as little irritability as possible, kindly remind the mind to stay. Bring your attention back to this vital breath. This seamless cycle of breathing in . . . and breathing out. Full inhalations . . . long exhalations . . .

When you're ready, gradually turn your inner attention out, make your mental awareness more physical, focus your mind on your body—head and neck, fingers and toes, arms and legs . . . As your inside world rejoins the outside world, it's only natural to open your eyes . . . to brighter lights, your present surroundings, and linger in this calmer, clearer, more self-compassionate state.

PRACTICE 14
Float—The Shorter Practice

Float is the shorter of the two formal breathing practices. Ideally, you will do the longer practice daily, as well as this shorter one, five minutes here, five minutes there. If you're thinking, "Gimme a break," I agree. You could use a break. And that's exactly what Float gives you—a five-minute breathing break—to take once or several times a day. If you can't spare five minutes or you have trouble sitting still, take five to meditate on the birds humming around the bird feeder, on the sunflowers swaying in the breeze, or on the steam rising from the soup pot. Short or long, formal or informal, it's all mindfulness practice. It's all beneficial.

Take a moment to make yourself comfortable and settle into a quiet breathing rhythm. With each cycle of breath, deepening the inhalation, lengthening the exhalation. Deeper, fuller inhalations . . . Longer, slower exhalations. (If you're well-acquainted with this practice, feel free to close your eyes at any point.)

On the next in-breath, take a deep, full breath, and hold it for a count of five. As you let it out, let it all the way out, and imagine floating on a raft of breath. On the in-breath, imagine or think about floating. On the out-breath

NO STUPID QUESTIONS

Q Soon after I start meditating, I fall asleep. How can I stay awake long enough to reap the benefits?

A If you're sleep-deprived, meditating for any length of time can knock you out faster than you can count a small herd of imaginary sheep. This is a good thing come bedtime, not so great during meditation practice. If you want the full benefit, you will need to be fully awake.

If you find yourself repeatedly falling asleep, definitely get a good night's sleep. Maybe consider practicing at a different time of day, or in a slightly less comfortable position. Generally, if you can graciously welcome sleepiness without giving in to it, this and the other potential practice crashers (boredom, impatience, worry) can become great teachers.

. . . away, away from the concerns of the day. On the in-breath, float. On the out-breath, care-free. Inhale: Float. Exhale: Away. Inhale: Float. Exhale: Free. Like a mantra: Float . . . Away . . . Float . . . Free . . .

If your mind starts drifting, bring it back to floating. If sensations or feelings pull your attention from its mooring, gently put it back on the breath and the words: Float . . . Away . . . Float . . . Free . . .

Focusing and refocusing on the raft of breath and the words until you can involve yourself more fully, and deeply, in floating.

After this practice comes to an end, use these words as a resource. Whenever you would like to feel lighter and more buoyant, inflate an imaginary raft and invite yourself to float . . . away . . . float . . . free . . . Bringing a greater sense of lightness and buoyancy with you now, as you gradually bring your awareness back to shore. Back to your surroundings. Back to the quiet calm of the present moment.

THE EATING PRACTICES

It's always useful to meditate on eating, but it's easier, at least initially, when you take charge of the setting, circumstances, and food. The easiest, most conducive setting is a quiet one, somewhere you can snack solo without distraction, or in the company of a mindful-eating friend or group. After you've tried these practices in the privacy of your kitchen, you might want to hone your new skill at a quiet café before you tackle an all-you-can-eat buffet in a noisy restaurant. Work up to more challenging dining situations over time. For now, turn off the TV, clear the table, and do whatever needs doing to set the stage for mindful eating.

You will also have an easier time of it if you try these eating practices when you are more than a little hungry, but not ravenous. For waist watchers who nourish themselves regularly over the course of the day, moderate hunger usually arises three to four hours after a meal. But if you're someone who routinely skips meals or eats skimpy meals, hunger may strike in an hour or two.

Finally, take it easy by starting with low-risk snacks, like raisins and whole-grain crackers, and working up to foods you're at the greatest risk of overeating.

While I suggest certain foods for certain practices, these are only suggestions. If you're on a calorie-restricted food plan, have other dietary restrictions, or just don't like the suggested food, feel free to substitute something similar. Whatever your food preferences, you may need to do a little food shopping. You'll find a shopping list at the top of those practices that require eating.

Ready to learn how to indulge your food cravings without overindulging?

PRACTICE 15
Mindless-Eating Meditation[2]

Shopping list: popcorn, freshly popped or store-bought

This is an exercise in mindless eating. Yes, you're about to mindlessly eat a handful of popcorn. Why? Because, when done carefully, mindless eating can be enlightening. If you're reluctant to make an intentional practice of mindless eating, not to worry. It's bound to happen unintentionally sooner or later. At which point, as soon as you notice yourself eating mindlessly, pay attention. Even if only for a few bites.

Before you grab a handful of popcorn, think about how our culture suggests we eat. How advertisers urge us to overindulge with slogans like, "Betcha can't eat just one." How our nearest and dearest coax us to overeat with their sincere, misguided pleas: "*Mangia, mangia,*" or "Clean your plate. Children are starving in India!" Take a moment to reflect before you intentionally do as they say, if not as they intend to do.

Popcorn ready?

Take a seat, but don't bother making yourself comfortable. Slump, lean . . . forget about good posture or breathing deeply. Take a few shallow breaths, or even better, intermittently hold your breath. Sitting like this makes everything worse. It strains your neck and back muscles, makes it difficult to relax or to concentrate. It's already more difficult to focus, isn't it? The more you think about your growing discomfort, the more difficult it gets. It's only a matter of time before boredom swoops in and your concentration plummets.

Ready or not, pick up a big handful of popcorn, or two; you've got two hands. Doesn't matter if you're hungry or if you even like popcorn. It's right here, in front of you; you might as well eat it. Eating is a great distraction. You could really use a distraction right about now. Why wait one more second? Start eating. Don't hold back. Wolf it down. Don't bother to taste or chew before swallowing. Eat as fast as you can. Shovel it in.

C'mon, hurry up. You've got a lot more to do today, you don't have time to eat. Better multitask. While you're eating, you could check your voicemail, read a magazine or watch TV. So much to do, so little time. If you hurry through this exercise, you can cross it off your to-do list. You've got errands to run, e-mails to answer, bills to pay. What about that doctor's appointment? Did you call to reschedule? Your to-do list is endless. Who's got time to eat mindfully? Getting to the supermarket is a stretch. You're dreaming if you expect to cook meals and eat them sitting down.

Okay, time to switch gears. If you haven't finished the popcorn, set it aside now. Take a deep breath, and let it out slowly. No more eating, just breathing. Slowing down, slowing way . . . down . . . And breathing fully, deeply, and slowly. Inviting yourself to notice how it feels to have eaten mindlessly: frantic, unsettling, confusing . . . Whatever you feel, feel it, acknowledge it, stay with it . . .

When you're ready, expand your awareness to include sensations—tension or relaxation, hunger or fullness—and

NO STUPID QUESTIONS

Q I've heard that breakfast is essential to permanent weight loss, but I'm not hungry when I roll out of bed. Should I force myself to eat something?

A While it's true that many a successful waist watcher eats a healthy breakfast, it doesn't mean *your* weight loss depends on consuming an early-morning meal. Rather than force-feeding yourself at the crack of dawn, consider waiting until you're mildly to moderately hungry (it'll happen eventually), and breaking the fast then.

thoughts, too. Noticing if you're judging yourself or beating yourself up for eating mindlessly, maybe eating more than you had intended. Bringing curiosity to your experience as it unfolds . . . to the feelings, sensations, and thoughts. To the natural rhythms of breathing. Deeper inhalations . . . Slower exhalations . . . Deeper . . . Slower . . .

As you continue to breathe, deeply, fully, take a few moments to reflect on this mindless-eating experience. Noticing your reactions, but taking no immediate action. Lingering, if you can, just a little longer in awareness, the foundation of lasting behavioral change.

PRACTICE 16
Hunger-Awareness Meditation

Dieting has made hunger an enemy, and the dieters who keep hunger at bay have become heroes and heroines in their daily battle of the bulge. Going hungry has become a point of pride, even when resisting hunger makes the hunger more persistent and insistent on your overeating. Many dieters have been so successful at estranging themselves from this basic instinct that they fail to recognize mild to moderate hunger. They know hunger only as ravenous.

This meditation shines the spotlight of awareness on physiological and emotional hunger, casting them in a warmer, truer light. Even if you're well acquainted with these fraternal twins, repeated practice will help you recognize and respond to them with greater care, wisdom, and skill.

Take a moment to make yourself comfortable, adjusting your position, loosening your belt, and making any other necessary adjustments. As the body settles into comfort, the breath naturally adopts a slower, quieter rhythm. The in-breath naturally deepening . . . the out-breath slowly lengthening. Breathing comfortably and rhythmically.

When you're ready, scan the body from head to toe, noticing areas of relaxation and tension, especially those areas that are barometers of your health and well-being. Pursuing neither comfort nor discomfort, just noticing sensations in the forehead, the face, the jaw. Moving your awareness down the neck and across the shoulders . . . Down the back to the lower back. Down to the belly and around the hips with minimal judgment, maximum self-compassion. Just noticing whatever you notice in, around, and throughout your body.

Inhaling, exhaling, and taking it from the top, scan the body for signs of physical hunger. Starting with the mind, notice your ability to concentrate. Assess if you're more interested in breathing or eating right now. Imagine what it would be like if a delicious meal suddenly appeared—how your eyes would respond to the color . . . your nose to the aroma . . . your taste buds to the taste. As you shine the spotlight of awareness on the stomach and around the abdomen, search like a detective for obvious clues and subtle hints. Do you detect a vague emptiness or something deeper, more cavernous? How about audible signals? Could that be a low rumble, a fierce growl? Keep imagining, sensing, listening for answers, collecting any and all clues to physical hunger.

Continuing to breathe, of course, naturally and steadily, as you do one last scan for emotional hunger signals. Without assuming or jumping to conclusions, check in with your feelings. Notice how you feel, and if you can, put a name to the feeling or mix of feelings. You probably know that some emotions, like irritability and crankiness, can be fueled by physical hunger. Others, like sadness and boredom, are more often a result of emotional hunger. Scan for the range of feelings without trying to change or suppress them. If you feel like eating, notice that, and ask yourself: "Am I hungry?" If there's little or no evidence of physical hunger, further your investigation. Ask yourself: "How do I really feel?" "What do I truly crave?" "Could I be emotionally hungry?" Keep breathing and noticing what helps you tell the difference between emotional and physical hunger. Remind

yourself that making important distinctions takes patience and practice. Repeated practice.

Practice that begins and ends with the breath. Deep inhalations, slow
exhalations. Quiet rhythms of breathing. Even if you now know you're
physically hungry, take a moment to quiet the mind, calm the body.
And when you feel complete, turn your inner attention to your outer
world, more aware of how you feel and what you need—even if what
you need is a little something, something that would really hit the spot.

PRACTICE 17
Taste-Satisfaction Meditation

Shopping list: A small box of raisins

When you're short on time, it's impractical to wait for your stomach's ultimate fullness signal, which comes fifteen to twenty minutes
too late. Too late for most waist watchers, who heed the signal only
as belated confirmation of what they already know—that they've
overeaten. If only you could get a quicker read on satisfaction so you
would clearly know when to put down your fork.

Happily, if you tune in to your taste buds' satiety signals, you can.
Not only do your taste buds give you the fastest, most accurate assessment of when you've eaten enough, they offer immediate feedback
on your eating pleasure and displeasure. These moment-by-moment
news bites help you answer questions you didn't know you had, like
"Is this meal worth finishing?"

Awareness of taste satiety or taste satisfaction can be cultivated
with just about any food—an orange, a Hershey's Kiss, even a potato
chip—but the raisin has become the hands-down favorite. No other
snack comes close to packing so much taste and texture into so few
calories. When you're ready (read: mildly to moderately hungry),
grab a napkin, three raisins, and take a seat.

Sitting with open eyes, make yourself comfortable, and take a few calming breaths. Full inhalations . . . long exhalations . . . Pick up one raisin and carefully inspect it as if it were your first. Notice the plumpness of this sun-dried grape, the intricacy of the folds, the variation in color. With the same curiosity, bring it under your nose and notice if there's an aroma and if you're salivating in anticipation. Place the raisin in your mouth and start chewing, noticing texture, taste, temperature. As you slowly chew, pay careful attention to your mouth's reaction, including the experience of your tongue and teeth. If thoughts or feelings pull your attention away, gently bring it back. Eating is the meditation. Allow yourself to enjoy eating without guilt or self-criticism. After all, you are nourishing your body. You are feeding yourself. Continue to chew purposefully . . . swallow intentionally. Fully appreciate the lingering taste of this first raisin.

When you're ready, pick up another raisin. Visually compare this one to the first—the size, the color, the moistness . . . Bring it under your nose, inhaling the aroma if there is one. Then pop this second raisin into your mouth and keep doing what you've been doing . . . eating mindfully. This time, notice the similarities and the differences. If you expected to enjoy the taste, notice if the second raisin meets your expectations, and how it compares to the first. Pay particular attention to the ever-changing experience of taste over time . . . taking all the time you need to savor, chew, swallow, and attend to any raisin goo stuck in your teeth.

When you're ready for the third raisin, invite yourself to mindfully eat it on your own. Of course, you can choose to stop at two, but if you want to learn more about taste satisfaction, proceed. You know the drill: notice whatever's noteworthy, especially how this raisin compares with the first two. If at any point you find yourself eating mechanically, automatically, inattentively, refocus on eating mindfully, purposefully, attentively. If judgment or self-criticism arises, acknowledge it, and refocus on mindfully eating this raisin. When you've finished swallowing the last bits, refocus on your body in the chair, sitting and breathing, deeply . . . fully . . . rhythmically. Imagine what would happen if you continued eating mindfully, even if it were just a little more mindfully, a little more often. Let yourself imagine how paying attention to the everyday act of eating might transform your eating habits, your weight-loss efforts, your life.

PRACTICE 18
Full-Body Fullness Scan

Shopping list: Whole-grain crackers, nut butter, or all-fruit jam

The taste buds may provide the quickest read on satiety, but when it comes to fullness, the human body works like the best cell phone on the clearest day. How's that? The body transmits a range of fullness signals—sensations, thoughts, and feelings—from head to toe.

Problem is, without an operator's manual, most adults don't know how to listen to their messages. We may be born with the ability to receive satiety's calls, but we quickly learn to screen them out. By the time new clients find my couch, they have disconnected from all but the most obvious signals, and have no idea how to reconnect. They're open to reestablishing a connection if it will help them lose weight, but they are unsure if they can, and clueless where to begin.

Think of this practice as the operator's manual you never got. First time through, you will get all the intellectual know-how you need in order to recognize the range of fullness cues. With repeated practice, you will develop enough self-confidence to respond to your personal cues in the best possible way—by reclaiming your innate ability to stop eating when you've had your fill.

To do this practice, you will need a tall glass of ice water and a large whole-grain cracker or several smaller ones, thinly smeared with your favorite nut butter or fruit spread. If you've got dietary restrictions or concerns, substitute any substantial, preferably high-fiber, snack.

Sitting with your snack within easy reach, make yourself comfortable and take a few calming breaths. Deepen the inhalation, lengthen the exhalation. Place one hand on the water glass, the other on your stomach. If you placed your hand below or on top of your belly button, move it up. The pear-shaped stomach lies between the belly button and the right breast. Invite yourself to drink as much water as you comfortably can, paying particular attention to the coolness as it travels down your throat and into your stomach. If you can feel the coolness in your stomach, focus on that. If you're aware of different sensations in and around your stomach, focus on those. You may notice a sense of filling up, a tightening of the waistband, a stretch across the abdomen. These are hallmarks of early fullness, but yours may differ. Give yourself permission to notice whatever you notice, attend to whatever needs attending. If you notice you're thirsty during this practice, be sure to quench your thirst.

Drink to your heart's content, then rest both hands by your side or in your lap. Clear the mind as you would cleanse the palate, using calming breaths like a spoonful of sorbet. As you continue to breathe, pick up the snack, letting the sight and smell help you anticipate the taste. Begin eating mindfully, focusing on your teeth's response to the texture, your tongue's take on the flavors, your whole mouth's reaction. Chewing slowly, intentionally, observe the unfolding experience of taste sensation. Without self-criticism or worry, permit yourself to enjoy the snack as long as you find it enjoyable. If you weren't all that hungry to start, you may notice taste quickly diminishing. If you're hungrier than you realized, the flavor may remain flavorful for many more bites. Setting aside assumptions, let your taste buds tell you when hunger fades into fullness.

After three or four bites, or as soon as you notice taste or flavor decreasing, shift your attention to your stomach and continue to eat. With attention tuned to sensations in the stomach and around the abdomen, you might notice your midsection is somewhat warmer, your waistband is a bit tighter, your stomach is slightly distended. You may experience some, all or none of these fullness signals. Initially, the signals can be unclear, confusing or seemingly nonexistent. Stay tuned. Notice whatever you notice, with as little judgment and self-criticism as possible.

If you run into mental static, notice the thoughts—the recriminations, rationalizations—and redirect your attention to the snack. If you encounter emotional static—boredom, worry, maybe irritation—observe the feelings, and refocus on tasting, chewing, savoring. Of course, you can choose to stop eating at any time. But if you have yet to detect comfortable fullness, eat some more, learn some more.

Invite yourself to expand your awareness, envelop your mind and body with gentle attention. Scanning from head to toe, notice your physical reaction to the food and drink you've consumed so far. If you're markedly fuller, you might notice that your mind has drifted from eating to other activities . . . that your eyes, nose, and tongue find the snack less appealing, less interesting . . . that your chewing pace has slowed down. You might not have noticed until now that your leg muscles are more supple, your feet are more restless, ready to move on. What you discover may surprise you.

Continue eating with careful attention until you experience a real change, a significant shift that indicates comfortable fullness. To get clear, you might ask yourself: "Do I feel satisfied?" "Am I full yet?" Whatever your answer, notice how you know what you know. If you remain uncertain, imagine how you might feel if you ate another cracker.

When most or all signs point to fullness, permit yourself to stop eating. If you're sure that you're full, but the eating urge remains, scan your body for feelings. Scanning from head to toe, do your best to name the feelings that might be fueling your urge to eat. Scanning, breathing, naming, then choosing. Yes, you can choose to keep eating to the point of physical discomfort, or you can find a way to emotionally comfort yourself. If you choose to overeat, continue to pay attention, to learn. For now. An hour from now. Through today, and into tomorrow.

However many bites you take, after you've taken the last bite, refocus on breathing—full inhalations, long exhalations—and appreciating what you're learning to do: discovering a kinder approach to sustainable weight loss by rediscovering your innate ability to recognize fullness.

PRACTICE 19
All-Purpose Eating Meditation, Part I
Shopping list: Six items on your risky food list [details below]

If you were to choose just one eating meditation for daily practice, this would be it. This ultimate practice combines all the meditations into one meditation. Before you make yourself comfortable and focus on the breath, wait up! To do this all-in-one exercise, you will need a risky food list that ranks foods according to your likelihood of overeating them. And you will likely need to go food shopping. Yes, I'm asking you to delay gratification, but it's for a worthy cause. You're not only preparing yourself for this meditation, you're developing a systematic plan for fear-free eating, a simple, all-purpose approach to mindful dining.

Mindful-eating training hasn't always been so systematic. In fact, yesteryear's programs scared off a lot of would-be participants by suggesting they savor whatever and however much they want. Understanding that dieters who have limited portion sizes since they were teenagers are terrified of sudden freedom, today's more scientific programs use risky food lists to help participants gradually face food fears.

PERSONAL SLIMMING LESSON

Join the Small Plate Club?

The size of your dinnerware affects the size of your appetite, food researchers have demonstrated, but does that mean you should join the small plate club? While studies have shown that individuals eat more when they're served more, it's unclear if they eat less when they serve *themselves* less. Before you start setting the table with doll-sized plates, why not investigate what a difference plate size makes to you?

Use nothing bigger than a salad plate for a day or two and see if serving yourself less does, in fact, cause you to eat less. Or, at the very least, reflect on snacks past. When you buy a 100-calorie snack pack, do you eat just one? When you serve yourself a small bowl of ice cream, do you go back for seconds? I usually do. Not because I'm hungry. No, it's more that I feel deprived. But that's just me.

Actually, it's my client Mary, too. To prevent herself from eating a second bowl, Mary lets her dog lick the first one clean. When her dog's loyal effort fails to curb her cravings, she digs directly into the carton and finishes the pint.

Do small plates work any better for you? If you would like to find out if reducing your plate size will shrink your waist size, look into it.

Why a risky food list? Because incrementally facing your fears is a tried-and-true strategy for overcoming them. Just ask a behavior therapist. When your fears are food-based, the mindful-eating plan begins with foods that pose little or no risk, then graduates to those you consider too risky to be near. When you can eat one serving of your highest-risk food with less fear, more confidence, you're good (or far better) to go wherever that food is served. But first you need a risky food list.

On the standardized risky food lists that mindful-eating groups use, raisins usually come before chocolate cake. That's because these lists are graded from least to most risky. Given that feared foods are so very personal, it's even more effective when you develop your personalized list. That way, you can incrementally confront the foods that trigger *your* overeating in the best possible order. If for example you consider chocolate cake a cakewalk, but raisins your downfall, it makes more sense to start with cake and finish with raisins. To help you understand the distinction between standardized and personalized lists, compare the two below.

Here's an example of a standardized list used in one mindful-eating training group:

Risky Food List

1. Risk free: raisins
2. Low risk: cheese & crackers
3. Moderate risk: chocolate snack-cake (e.g., Hostess Ho-Hos)
4. Higher risk: chips
5. Much higher risk: pot-luck meal
6. Highest risk: all-you-can-eat buffet

This is my personalized list:

Risky Food List

1. Risk free: vanilla yogurt
2. Low risk: crystallized ginger
3. Moderate risk: Hershey's Milk Chocolate Kisses
4. Higher risk: chips & salsa
5. Much higher risk: General Tso's chicken
6. Highest risk: Häagen-Dazs dulce de leche ice cream

Now it's your turn. In making your risky food list, keep in mind that the best lists feature a variety of foods, ranging from low- to high-risk. Not every last temptation.

Risky Food List

1. Risk free: _____

2. Low risk: _____

3. Moderate risk: _____

4. Higher risk: _____

5. Much higher risk: _____

6. Highest risk: _____

PRACTICE 20

All-Purpose Eating Meditation, Part II

Like saying grace, practicing this mealtime meditation enhances awareness and appreciation of the eating experience. Ideally, you will make the items on your risky food list the object of six sequential meditations. After that, you can focus the same mindful awareness on home-cooked meals and restaurant dinners. Snacks, too. Realistically, do what you're ready, willing, and able to do.

To start, practice the six sequential meditations on six separate occasions. On the first occasion, you will meditate on the first food. On the second, you will focus on the second. Practice session by practice session, you will munch your way down the list until on the sixth go-round, when you will mindfully eat the sixth item. No need to stop at six. Beef up your risky food list and keep practicing one item at a time until you feel confident enough to meditate on a simple meal.

If a particular list item causes you undue anxiety, do what you can to reduce your anxiety and increase your confidence beforehand. Consider doing one or more of the following: practicing when you're not too hungry; buying an individual serving; enlisting a mindful-eating buddy. There's definitely safety in numbers. If you don't trust yourself to keep all the foods in your cupboard, consider buying one at a time. If it turns out you can't stop yourself from overeating a feared item, take additional precautions, and try again later.

One final precaution: This all-purpose script is purposefully short. It doesn't give you the kind of bite-by-bite guidance you have come to expect from previous practices. Instead, it prompts you to do what you've been learning to do—pay gentle attention to the eating experience from start to finish. In other words, don't rush to finish the last bite by script's end. Keep the prompts in mind as you sit down to mindfully eat whatever you're eating, but take all the time you need.

Take a comfortable seated position and a few calming breaths, focusing on the word "ease" as you exhale. For the full length of each exhalation, silently repeat "eeeaaase." As you continue to lengthen the exhalation and deepen the inhalation, do three quick scans. One: scan the body for comfort, noticing areas that are more and less comfortable. Two: scan for hunger, noticing the range of physical hunger signals from subtle to obvious. Three: scan for emotional hunger, searching for feelings that might be fueling your urge to eat. Then adjust accordingly. If you're physically uncomfortable, make yourself more comfortable. If you're hungry, but not necessarily for food, check in with your feelings. Are there any emotional adjustments you need to make? If you're hungry, truly hungry, the only adjustment left to make is to shift your attention to the food before you.

When it makes sense, begin eating mindfully, paying particular attention to taste. If the taste is pleasurable, permit yourself the pleasure of eating. Tasting, enjoying, attending to the inevitable decrease in taste sensation, the eventual increase in the satisfaction of your taste buds, stomach fullness, and other hallmarks of fullness. If there's mental static, notice what you're thinking and refocus on eating. If there's emotional static, consider how you feel, what you need, and if you need to keep eating. If you're unsure, take a few more bites and reassess.

If it keeps making sense, keep eating, ever-attentive to personal hints and global signals of comfortable fullness—a sense of well-being, relaxation, ease. When you've had your fill, take a refreshing

breath and a quiet moment to reflect on your eating experience
before easing on to whatever's next.

The saying may be, "Practice makes perfect," but the goal of mindful-
eating practice is clearly not perfection. You can aim for perfection—to
savor each and every bite—as long as you also work toward accepting and welcoming imperfection. You're human, don't forget. Human
beings frequently miss the mark. You might do better with a more
realistic goal, like bringing mindful attention to however many bites
of however many meals as you can. You will definitely do better with a
self-compassionate attitude however mindfully or mindlessly you eat.
You might do best with a small, short-term goal, say, committing for
a few weeks to breathe when you breathe, taste when you taste, chew
when you chew, notice what you notice. Then retake this chapter's
quiz. Your new, improved score will help you rediscover two simple
truths about mindfulness practice: you don't have to be perfect, and
you don't have to practice for a lifetime to change for good.

PART IV

Social Support

*The Power of
Compassionate
Community*

THE SUCCESSFUL
WEIGHT-LOSS BUDDY

The more I help others to succeed, the more I succeed.

RAY KROC

Most people don't want to believe that when it comes to permanent weight loss, you gotta have social support. Whether that support comes from a diet club, therapy group, health-care institution, or a small circle of friends, you need some number of somebodies behind you. Or at least one weight-loss buddy.

I nod knowingly when new clients tell me they would prefer to avoid scrutiny and embarrassment by keeping their weight-loss efforts secret. I understand. I used to shy away from support groups myself. Although, like many clients, I wouldn't have been caught dead at a Weight Watchers meeting, I had no problem following the diet on my own. (That is, for the week or two I could stick to it.)

Because I do understand, I don't lecture clients on the measurable difference social support makes to health, happiness, and habit change. Nor do I insist they join a weight-loss group. Instead, I review the options—familiar self-help groups like Overeaters Anonymous, commercial organizations such as Weight Watchers, as well as less familiar options in the community and on the Internet—including therapy groups, restaurant-based slimming clubs, diet-betting web-sites (where dieters can bet on their future success), and chat rooms. You know, those real-time online coffee klatches.

I also share stories and recommend reading on the transformative power of social support. One such book is *Pack of Two* by the late author Caroline Knapp.[1] After a long, lonely battle with anorexia and alcoholism, Knapp found inner strength with the help of her beloved dog Lucy and Alcoholics Anonymous, among other supports. Only when clients are ready do I encourage them to find strength and com-passion in numbers.

That said, I *will* encourage you to dive into this chapter. I realize that social support doesn't have the magical allure of hypnosis, the Eastern appeal of meditation, the je ne sais quoi of self-compassion. The phrase "social support" has more of an off-putting effect. Just the word "support," for many veteran dieters, has become synonymous with social awkwardness, public humiliation, and certain failure. I will tell you, however, that what you're about to learn will expand the idea of social support, if not challenge long-standing assumptions and lead to new, unexpected conclusions.

I will also introduce you to community members who have succeeded beyond their wildest weight-loss dreams. Like Alex, an obese business-man who lost 160 pounds, halving his body weight, with a lot of help from his friends. It isn't that much of a surprise, considering what sci-entific minds have discovered about unified efforts. Are you aware, for example, that group therapy produces greater weight loss than indi-vidual therapy, even among clients who say they prefer the undivided attention of an individual therapist? Weight loss, researchers have reason to believe, is positively contagious. Their eye-opening research findings are the kind that inspire waist watchers to buy memberships and other impulse purchases they will never use. Best to slow down long enough to learn basic concepts, the best options. The lingo, too.

WHO YOU GONNA CALL?

There are lots of definitions of social support, and many have to do with who you gonna call in a crisis? Who is going to catch you when you fall on physical, emotional, or financial hard times? While the friends and family who make up your human safety net can be life-savers, they can't necessarily save you from overdosing on pepperoni pizza. In fact, some of your best allies in a life catastrophe can be your worst enemies in your personal weight-loss battle.

So who you gonna call for weight-loss support? Jenny Craig? Your partner in overeating? Fido? If the very question inspires more despair than hope, you've got plenty of company. Even clients who long for community have been known to respond to the who-you-gonna-call question with some variation of "I'd rather do it myself." There's ample reason why waist watchers fail to embrace support groups. If you've had negative experiences, you've probably got a few reasons of your own. If your experience was particularly painful, you might be asking yourself the question that rugged individualists like author Ayn Rand made their name asking: Collective effort, what is it good for? It's a good question. I encourage you to keep it in mind as you read on.

Generally, the term "social support" refers to people helping people. More specifically, there's positive social support, a conscious and generous act committed by those who encourage others to meet goals. There's also negative support, that thing some people do, often subconsciously, when they discourage healthy change. Like when someone buys a waist watcher the very snack she's sworn off, or insists on eating the sworn-off snack in her company.

Social support is a measurable concept with quantifiable benefits. Researchers have developed standardized tests to assess the quantity (how many people) and quality (how personally satisfying) of an individual's support system. (Quality, more than quantity, is a stronger predictor of good things to come.) With these scales, countless researchers have counted the ways social support benefits the health and well-being of such diverse populations as pregnant women, breast cancer survivors, diabetics, cardiac patients, and yes, waist watchers.[2] Whether or not you agree with Barbra Streisand—that people who need people are the luckiest people—there's much to be gained by assessing your support network, then strengthening it if need be. (In the next chapter, you will get the chance to assess the strength of your current network.)

For now, it's worth remembering that you are no stranger to support. You started this life in groups (family, school, church), and you live as well as you do because of various collective efforts (community, work, government). We are undeniably social creatures, and we generally do better when we are surrounded by a herd of creatures who love, support, and encourage us.

From day one of human history, social support has proven enormously helpful. First and foremost, for survival. In the beginning, early men and women banded together to hunt, gather, and ward off wooly mammoths. Centuries later, when our primitive predecessors moved into town and got more civilized, they worked shoulder to shoulder on higher purposes, like liberty, justice, and human welfare. But it wasn't until the twentieth century that groups purposefully gathered for therapeutic purposes.

MISERY LOVES COMPANY?

Historians single out a Boston doctor named Joseph Pratt as the innovator of group therapy. With tuberculosis cases on the rise back in 1905, it made good, practical sense for Pratt to teach his TB patients about the deadly disease en masse. But the idea of therapy groups had been brewing since the late 1800s, when settlement houses were founded to help America's burgeoning immigrant population find work and shelter. Another turn-of-last-century health-care provider who gets a nod for prescribing the talking cure collectively is a disciple of Sigmund Freud's, Alfred Adler. Unlike Freud, who understood psychological problems to reside in an individual's psyche, Adler's understanding of psychic pain took into account his patients' social circles.

To be fair, credit for group therapy's skyrocketing popularity belongs to a number of health professionals, notably Irvin Yalom, the psychiatrist and group-therapy scholar, and Aaron Beck, the forefather of cognitive therapy. Nonprofessionals, too: two names that stand out are Bill Wilson, cofounder of Alcoholics Anonymous, and Jean Nidetch, innovator of Weight Watchers.

When I talk about group therapy, I am talking in the broadest possible sense about any group of any size that works toward the social, psychological, or behavioral change of its members. I am talking about the range of offerings, from an exclusive, deluxe, multisession weight-loss program taught by an elite team of psychologists, nutritionists, and exercise physiologists, to a free, introductory mindful-eating workshop offered by one meditation enthusiast. If I had to speak more definitively, choose one defining characteristic, it wouldn't be the frequency or location of group meetings, but the common purpose of its members.

More than individual contributions, economic trends have made group therapy what it is today—the most widely used treatment mode. Half a century ago, groups popped up wherever and whenever the demand for services outweighed the supply of individual therapists, including prisons, mental hospitals, and child-guidance centers. But with the astronomic rise of health-care costs, the advent of managed care, and the ever-increasing use of the Internet for health information, groups have become as plentiful and accessible as Facebook friends.

Today it's not unusual for group therapy to be prescribed instead of individual counseling. For two reasons: it's at least as effective *and* it costs less. According to more than seven hundred studies, therapy delivered in a group format has a consistent and positive effect on the range of physical and mental health complaints. When group therapy is successful, as it is in 85 percent of the cases, members report a greater sense of self-awareness and self-acceptance, and a stronger sense of belonging. In other words, group-goers stand to gain more self-compassion than individual clients.[3]

Guys like Mark, a recovering compulsive overeater who once tipped the scales at 365 pounds, are living proof that group therapy is generally more beneficial than individual. Looking back over three-plus decades of psychotherapy, Mark credits his lasting success to the ongoing support of Overeaters Anonymous (OA). Like dieting, attending individual therapy helped Mark temporarily change his eating habits and his appearance, but the man himself remained unchanged. Telling psychotherapists what he thought they wanted to hear—essentially "I'm OK, you're OK"—it was only a matter of time before he would regain what he lost. As Mark sees it now, his recovery began when he met his match at OA. "Group members call you on what you're saying," he explains. "More truth comes out." And more weight stays off. Mark, who now weighs a healthy 210 pounds, has maintained a 155-pound weight loss for going on twenty years. In other words, when he stopped fooling health-care providers, among other supporters, he could honestly start taking care of himself.

JOIN ANY CLUB?

In thinking about weight-loss groups, the main distinction is between therapy groups and support groups, also known as self-help groups. All groups share an interest in helping members decrease suffering and isolation, increase resilience and a sense of belonging, but what separates therapy from support groups is leadership and ideology. Therapy groups are guided by psychological theory and the health-care professionals who run them. Support groups are less driven by theoretical perspective, less dependent on professional leadership, and are just as likely to be led by veteran members as by licensed practitioners.

Traditional therapy groups are a microcosm of real-life relationships, providing members with an opportunity to confront long-standing interpersonal issues in the relative safety of their therapist's office. Of course, weight-loss support groups are microcosms, too. After all, everyone travels through life carrying some amount of interpersonal baggage. But weight-loss groups focus on weight loss, not relationship issues, and are therefore nothing like the off-putting stereotypes portrayed in movies like *One Flew Over the Cuckoo's Nest*. More like energizing health classes than emotional family reunions, support groups for the range of eating issues focus more on thoughts and behaviors than feelings. Some groups, like those for people with eating disorders, may encourage members to share feelings, but as a rule, most concern themselves with the thoughts that trigger overeating episodes and the behaviors that help prevent them.

If you were to eavesdrop on a typical weight-loss group, you would hear talk of "self-monitoring" or how to keep food journals, weight graphs, and other personal records to track progress and regress. You might also hear mention of other cognitive-behavioral therapy concepts, like "stimulus control," which is delivering yourself from temptation by, among other things, ditching the Doritos and Cheez Whiz and restocking the cupboards with healthier snacks; "cognitive restructuring," which is rewriting erroneous thoughts that make ordering a venti mochaccino with extra whipped cream sound like a good source of calcium; and "relapse prevention," which are proven strategies for wearing the same sized jeans year after year. Group leaders might also talk about savoring each bite and other mindful-eating principles. A few groups might suggest members adopt a very low-calorie diet for quick weight loss (and, sadly, rapid regain), but most would recommend good nutrition over rigid dieting.

When groups are effective, the entity is larger than the sum of its individual members. This truism holds true for all kinds of groups, agree members who have tried a number of different groups and researchers who have studied the effectiveness of various group treatments. But to the Groucho Marxes of the world, the mountain of irrefutable evidence doesn't amount to a hill of beans. Skeptics of therapy groups can't imagine how the blind leading the blind could go anywhere but astray. That commiserating could be curative strikes critics as not only illogical, but inconceivable.

CHANGE FOR THE BETTER?

Yet there's good reason to believe that groups cure. In what has become the bible on group therapy, Irvin Yalom's *Theory and Practice of Group Psychotherapy*, the scholarly psychiatrist cites eleven good reasons or "curative factors." The three top reasons: hope, universality, and altruism. Groups work, Yalom writes, because for one, they instill *hope*. There's something about meeting people who have been successful that inspires the thought: "Gee, if she could do it, maybe I can." Secondly, hearing how members struggle in similar ways reminds individual group-goers that they are surely not alone, that there's a *universality* to suffering. Finally, the giving-and-taking characteristic of groups rewards each member with a greater sense of *altruism*.[4] From this more optimistic, interconnected, compassionate place, change happens.

Over the sixteen to twenty-four weeks of a standard weight-loss therapy, participants predictably change physically and psychologically. Psychologically, members experience a greater sense of well-being, evidenced in lower scores on depression tests and higher marks on measures of self-esteem and body image. Physically, the average member bids a fond farewell to 7–10 percent of her body weight. A good number also say good-bye to high blood pressure, elevated cholesterol levels, and other indices of poor health, if not hasta la vista to the medications previously prescribed to keep those conditions in check. Because the most dramatic changes happen in the first four to six months, some groups try to make maximum change in minimum time with very low-calorie menus or meal-replacement products. As I have mentioned, these calorically challenged treatments enable participants to lose more initially and regain more rapidly.[5]

Groups that prescribe very low-calorie diets aren't the only ones that set members up for regain. All weight-loss groups have a better track record with weight loss than maintenance. Members of Weight Watchers, for example, lose 5.3 percent of their body weight the first year, but by the second year, that initial weight loss dwindles to 3.2 percent. (Members who lose and maintain the most, no surprise, are those who attend the most meetings.) With an initial weight loss of 7–10 percent, participants in short-term therapy groups, on average, do significantly better than commercial diet group-goers. However, they too subsequently regain a third of what they lose.[6]

THREE STEPS TO SUCCESS

I cite these statistics not to bring you down, but to wake you up. Clearly, weight-loss groups could learn a few things about sustainable weight loss. We all can. But some long-term groups and individual waist watchers have learned to maintain weight loss for a year, two, three, and more. To understand the secret to their success, researchers have spent decades studying these exceptional individuals and groups. Extensive media coverage of key research findings has made some of their personal habits common knowledge. Most of them eat breakfast and exercise an hour a day, and weigh themselves once a week. But three secrets have remained relatively hidden in the social support studies.

Secret one: Invest in support. It may not be absolutely, positively essential, but a little support can make a big difference on the bathroom scale. (Take it from successful waist watchers who have joined the National Weight Control Registry. That's the national database of more than five thousand individuals who have lost and maintained the loss of an average of 66 pounds for five and a half years. While registration requires members to maintain a 30-pound weight loss for at least a year, the Registry's greatest successes have lost as many as 300 pounds. Of these enviable successes, it's worth noting that 55 percent say they couldn't have done it without a nutritionist, a doctor, a self-help group—some kind of support.[7] Rather than buying one more diet book or exercise gadget, you might want to consider investing (or reinvesting) in your support network.

Secret two: Stay in touch. It's easy enough to find a short-term therapy group, but not a long-term one. Clients and therapists just aren't that into them. Programs that exceed twenty weeks are expensive, and suffer from a high dropout rate. Yet when it comes to weight maintenance, members of long-term programs who maintain contact with treatment providers fare far better than those who lose touch after attending a short-term group. Clients who attend weekly sessions for six months typically maintain 50–60 percent of their initial weight loss. Tack on another six to twelve months of additional therapist contact as state-of-the-art weight-loss programs do, and participants maintain a whopping 80–100 percent.[8] Staying in touch, it seems, helps waist watchers navigate the inevitable obstacles and stay the course.

Professional contact (with a psychotherapist, a doctor, a nutritionist) appears superior to nonprofessional (a sponsor, a support-group leader), but researchers can't be sure. The anonymity of members who belong to Overeaters Anonymous and some of the other nonprofessional groups makes them all but impossible to study. Nevertheless, the anecdotal evidence of these groups is promising, and the price is surely right. Self-help groups offer lifetime support at little or no cost. The jury may still be out, but the verdict is fairly certain: for weight maintenance, ongoing support makes a world of difference.

Secret three: Catch some enthusiasm. Before you jump to quotable conclusions—that it takes a village to achieve sustainable weight loss—take a deep breath. All that's really required is one successful partner. Study subjects who teamed up with at least one weight-loss success (someone who lost 10 percent of their body weight) lost significantly more weight over the course of eighteen months than subjects with one or more unsuccessful partners, or no partner at all.[9]

Slimness is proving to be as contagious as the common cold, assert social scientists Nicholas Christakis and James Fowler. Obesity, too. If you're having trouble losing weight, look around. Your friends might be making you fat, suggest the scientists and coauthors of *Connected*, their book on social networks.[10] In fact, simply sitting next to an overeater appears to up your odds of overeating.

FINDING THINSPIRATION

Dine with a Mindful Eater

When I'm low on mindful-eating inspiration, I can always refuel at Alice's. Not the restaurant, mind you, but the cozy kitchen of my dear friend and mindful-eating colleague Alice Rosen. Winter, spring, summer, or fall, I can always find this creative cook whipping up something tasty and nourishing, if not inspiring. But never intentionally low-cal. Calories are beside the point when there's a chill in the air and Alice ladles you a mug of hot cocoa with vanilla marshmallows or a goblet of her mother's whipped eggnog.

Come grill season, meals at Chez Alice are naturally lower in calorie and often alfresco. Under a mosquito net and the aromatic canopy of pine trees, Alice has been known to turn dinner into a cinematic production. Picture Meryl Streep eating under the stars in *Out of Africa*. Some enchanted fall evening, Alice retreats to the living room, where she stokes up the hardwood stove, brings out the cloth napkins, and lays out a sumptuous spread of seasonal appetizers. On one memorable occasion, "sumptuous" was a gingery eggplant spread on whole-grain crackers with a beautiful assortment of multicolored cherry tomatoes.

Dinner with Alice reliably reminds me that food nourishes the body AND the soul. That eating is a sensual delight, a cause for celebration, an open invitation to practice mindfulness. Need a helping of inspiration? Invite a mindful eater to lunch. Or better yet, send out an Evite for a mindful potluck.

The social contagion theory of human behavior helps explain the incredible success of waist watchers like Alex, the businessman who halved his body weight attending OA meetings with guys like Mark. Inspired by Alex's success, a dozen of his nearest and dearest, including his son the ice-cream maker, have also met success. "We all have one thing in common," Alex e-mailed, "we continue to work the program." That, and they continue to enjoy good, supportive company.

Social contagion also sheds light on the yo-yoing weight of veteran dieters like Oprah, who began climbing toward inexorable weight gain on her big cross-country eating adventure. For eleven days in 2006, the well-intentioned talk show host and her friend Gayle were partners in overindulgence. Had Oprah driven the 3,600 miles with her personal trainer or one of her favorite medical consultants, would she have forgone the biscuits and apple butter? The cheeseburgers and fries? Hard to say, but odds are she would have indulged in smaller portions.

If you're interested in catching the sustainable weight-loss bug, you're in luck. The opportunity for finding like-minded waist watchers has never been greater, especially if you've got Internet access. Whether you live in the heart of a thriving metropolis, at a great distance from civilization, or somewhere in between, you can now access support 24–7 if you've got a computer with a connection. This is good news, especially for those who are physically disabled or otherwise less than mobile.

Getting to your biggest and best supporters without getting overwhelmed is the trick. To that end, I have organized the big buffet of support options into bite-sized sections, and I have reviewed the advantages and disadvantages of each. The menu items, you'll soon see, fall into two columns: (A) in-person, and (B) online communities. And several subcategories of professional and nonprofessional support. By professional, I mean guidance offered by licensed health-care providers. By nonprofessional, I'm talking about groups that require no particular fancy initials (PhD, MD, LICSW, RN) nor theoretical perspective of their leaders.

By way of previewing the upcoming review: if you make only one choice, choose one from column A, not B, if you can. Why's that? Because waist watchers who attend actual groups typically lose more weight than those who log on to virtual networks. If your only option is virtual, not to worry. You can still meet success connecting with at least one successful virtual weight-loss buddy.

In all honesty, I am not advocating one group over another. I have done my mindful best to stick to the facts, citing current research and client experience throughout. Sure, I've got my favorites, but my preferences are just that: my preferences. As you sample the menu, see which one(s) seem most satisfying. These are the ones you will want to consider as a regular source of sustenance.

In-Person Support
Nonprofessional Support

Every year, millions of dieters join Weight Watchers and other non-professional support groups, and some dieters meet some amount of success. It's hard to say exactly how many meet how much success, because federal law doesn't require weight-loss organizations to see the error or the efficacy of their ways. Until recently, if you wanted to find an effective weight-loss program, you would have done just as well playing eeny-meeny-miny-mo as trying to make an intelligent choice.

Comparison shopping got a little easier in 2005, when a respected team of researchers synthesized the existing evidence for the first major review of American weight-loss programs. Because of the paucity of solid scientific research, this major reexamination of the most popular plans didn't pick a winner, but it did point out the most and least promising. Below, I've summed up their key findings on commercial and self-help plans.[11]

Besides a financial interest in their membership, the big three commercial plans—Weight Watchers, Jenny Craig, and LA Weight Loss—have three things in common: a minimally trained, nonprofessional staff; a moderately restricted diet; and a modicum of behavioral counseling. All three also sell food products, but only Jenny provides packaged entrees as part of the package deal. The simplicity of a limited menu and the convenience of prepared food appeals to busy dieters who fantasize about hiring a personal chef. When holidays and vacations roll around, sticking to the plan gets more complicated and less convenient, even for the most dedicated customer who willingly packs her suitcases with these packaged foods. For most waist watchers, these foods may seem like the answer to their prayers, but more often than not, they turn out to be just another false hope.

The big three also have big differences. First and foremost, Weight Watchers is the only program with solid science behind it. Jenny Craig and LA Weight Loss have yet to put their diets to the scientifically rigorous test. Weight Watchers is also the only plan to provide living, breathing community in large groups; the other two serve up support individually. Members who have Internet access *can* find virtual community in chat rooms facilitated by Jenny Craig and Weight Watchers, but not LA Weight Loss. Cost is the ultimate differentiator: Weight Watchers is far more affordable ($10–12 per week in 2010) than Jenny Craig ($70–100). Trying to find the LA Weight Loss price tag is like locating a contact lens in a Jacuzzi.

Like commercial diet organizations, nonprofit weight-loss groups—Overeaters Anonymous (OA) and Take Off Pounds Sensibly (TOPS)—are also run by laypeople, often veteran members who have wrestled with their own eating problems. And neither can point to recent or accurate research on the effectiveness of their approach. The big difference between the commercial and not-for-profit groups is the price they place on membership: both OA and TOPS provide support at little or no cost.

The main distinction between the two self-help groups is their treatment philosophy. TOPS, like Weight Watchers, prescribes a modest low-cal diet, weekly weigh-ins, and real-life group support, and teaches a standard curriculum on diet, exercise, and behavior modification. More like Alcoholics Anonymous than any of the other weight-loss programs, Overeaters Anonymous takes a more complex view of the problem that brings members to meetings, and offers a more ambitious solution. In OA's view, behind every eating problem, from obesity to anorexia, is a problematic relationship with feelings (sadness, loneliness, anger, and so forth). OA's solution or resolution to both eating and feeling problems is a twelve-step plan that guides members toward physical, emotional, and spiritual recovery.

I know I've been saying that diets don't work, and yet Overeaters Anonymous has perfected the support piece. Remember Mark, the client unchanged by therapy but transformed by OA, who has maintained a 155-pound weight loss for going on two decades? Well, he has found compassionate community in meetings across America, as well as in Nairobi, Jerusalem, and Paris. Because the character of OA groups can vary widely, would-be members are encouraged to sample a variety of meetings, and freely interpret OA's spiritual notion of a "higher power." While some can't quite wrap their minds around the idea, those who can believe that, more than the group meetings and eating guidelines (no longer officially distributed but still available unofficially by selct groups), the empowering support they get from their higher power is the real secret to success.

Professional Support

Like ice cream, therapy groups come in many great flavors. You've no doubt heard of, if not tasted, some of the more popular choices—psycho-dynamic, cognitive-behavioral, and mindfulness-based psychotherapy. But maybe you're unaware of the shared ingredient between all of them: professional leadership. Back in Freud's day, psychodynamic theories were all the rage in individual and group therapy. Early therapy-goers were encouraged to review past troubles for unconscious clues to present-day problems. Today, the theory of choice, at least for weight-loss groups, is cognitive-behavioral therapy (CBT). More than childhood issues, CBT clients generally concern themselves with more pressing concerns. More specifically, rather than exploring shared, entrenched relationship difficulties like psychodynamic group members do, CBT group-goers find new and better ways of coping with common problems.

CBT groups are generally a short-term investment, meeting sixty to ninety minutes weekly or every other week, for four to six months. Held in a variety of settings (mental health centers, hospitals, therapy offices) membership costs about one-third to one-half of individual therapy, if that. Insurance often covers some, if not all of the fee ($40–$60 per session).

Adult waist watchers, you're learning, do well in CBT groups, but children do even better. Overweight kids who have joined a family-based slimming group weighed in significantly lighter than their solitary peers, even ten years afterward.[12] People who attend CBT groups for eating disorders also make good progress. Binge eaters who have joined a CBT group, in fact, have made measurably more progress than bingers involved in a self-help group.[13]

In the last decade, mindfulness-based therapy groups have become an increasingly popular treatment choice for the range of eating issues. Attendance is up in mindful-eating groups because they have helped members do what many dare not dream: enjoy eating without over-eating. These groups, originally developed as a cost-efficient treatment for eating disorders, are also proving to be an effective treatment for "eating disturbances," everyday eating problems that fall short of life-threatening disorders.

Just ask Cathy, a thirty-seven-year-old marketing director and self-proclaimed mindless snacker, who took my crash course in Mindfulness-Based Eating Awareness Training. "If I had read about mindful eating in a magazine, I don't know if I would have implemented it," Cathy says. "But with a group, it's like working out with a personal trainer. You just do it." And "it" starts paying off almost immediately. Making mindfulness a team effort, this stressed-out exec worked meditation into her busy schedule and decreased her stress and stress-induced snacking in just five sessions.

While nutrition groups are more educational than psychotherapeutic, they are definitely supportive. Discussion may lean toward low-density calories and high-quality carbohydrates, but the better groups also discuss psychological slimming strategies. Run by registered dietitians, licensed nurses, and other health professionals, nutrition groups meet in a variety of settings—private nutrition practices, hospitals, universities. Some, not all, are covered by health insurance. If money's tight, it's possible to earn and learn by joining a weight-loss study at an academic institution involved in nutrition research, such as the Human Nutrition Research Center on Aging at Boston's Tufts University.

In study after study, group treatment has proven at least as effective as individual therapy. But for waist watchers, the end result is worth repeating, bold-facing, and italicizing. *Even for individuals who prefer one-on-one counseling, group therapy is proving superior.* In one study, group members lost 11 percent of their body weight, out-performing individual therapy-goers by 2 percent. The 9 percent that individual clients lost is nothing to sneeze at, mind you, but in weighing your support options, that 2 percent is worth keeping in mind.[14] That said, let me state the obvious: statistics are tidy averages that aren't meant to reflect individual differences or real-life circumstances. For waist watchers in the throes of a life crisis or a serious mental-health issue, individual therapy makes more sense.

NO STUPID QUESTIONS

Q The only thing listening to dieters whine about weight ever inspired me to do was to overeat. Given my negative reaction to diet groups, wouldn't I be better off on my own?

A I hope you know you're far from the only one who finds traditional diet-group discussions off-putting, if not counter-productive. I do, too. And yet I don't think you're better off alone. You'd do better to get support from a less traditional group of like-minded waist watchers.

To help you figure out who might be better, ask yourself three questions: Who's previously inspired you to lose weight (athletes, health-care professionals, colleagues)? Is there an existing group that attracts or is led by such inspirational figures? If not, have you considered teaming up with one or more motivated friends, colleagues, or relatives? If answers don't immediately spring to mind, keep asking and you shall receive.

Before undergoing stomach-reduction surgery, the personal attention of an individual therapist made a lot more sense than yet another diet for Edie. Remember Edie? She's the gastric-bypass patient from chapter 5, who modeled her new, petite shape in a little black dress. Before she could meet success and a group she could call her own, this fifty-seven-year-old travel agent had tried and failed with several weight-loss groups. Not because she was lazy or any of the other less than compassionate reasons discouraged dieters like Edie imagine. No, before this discouraged dieter could meet success, she needed help crawling out from under a major depression, a dead-end job, and a difficult family situation.

"If I didn't do individual therapy first," Edie says, "I absolutely wouldn't have had the courage [to undergo surgery]." Seventy-five pounds physically and emotionally lighter, she's graduated from weekly individual therapy sessions to a monthly support group for post-surgical patients. Between the real encouragement she gets from the hospital staff and group members, and the virtual support she finds on websites like obesityhelp.com, Edie remains hopeful and motivated. She is intent on keeping off what she has lost, and working on losing more.

CREATE-YOUR-OWN SUPPORT

You're in luck if you can find an existing weight-loss group to meet all or most of your needs, but what if you're not so lucky? You could do what a lot of waist watchers do—do it yourself. Forge ahead solo. Or, knowing that social support is one of the most powerful predictors of long-term success, you could create your own support. Like what? With whom? Good questions! To help you find your own satisfying answers, consider the surprising results research psychologists and creative waist watchers have discovered about different group efforts.

If you've got a significant other, and you're both overweight, it may seem like a winning proposition to team up and slim down together. In a comprehensive review of a dozen weight-loss studies, the joint effort of spouses can and has been shown to work better than solo attempts. At least for a few months.[15] But, as you may have learned from personal experience, teaming up with your partner can backfire too, especially if he or she doesn't share your enthusiasm. Or if your significant other has been known to bring home the very treat you're trying to avoid. Weight gain, it's worth remembering, can be just as contagious as weight loss. I've never calculated the number of clients who have told me their most significant weight gain began soon after meeting their significant other, but I trust I would run out of fingers and toes long before I finished calculating.

When it comes to weight maintenance, a small circle of friends beats a romantic partnership and a party of one. That's the general consensus among researchers, including the authors of the landmark study on peer support, which compared solitary waist watchers with groups of four friends. More than the individual waist watchers, the friend teams proved more successful at sticking with the program, losing weight, and keeping it off. Six months after completing the friendly comparison, two-thirds of the team players, but only one-quarter of the singletons, were as slim as the day they graduated.[16]

Which doesn't mean your biggest supporters will be dear friends, but not your dearly beloved. Sometimes a combined effort is most effective. Take inspiration from a mother of two who once tipped the scales at 190 pounds. When her youngest left for college, this empty nester adopted two health-mates: her overweight husband and an energetic colleague. With her husband, she enjoyed cooking up lighter versions of their favorite recipes. With her high-energy colleague, she had fun exploring New England back roads by road bike. By the time the next academic year rolled around, this happier homemaker had pedaled one thousand miles and reached a healthy 145 pounds. Compared to the big self-help groups that had previously helped her lose weight but never maintain a comparable weight loss, this little group effort feels more sustainable because it's far more pleasurable and personal. "I don't feel deprived," she says. "I've made eating healthy and losing weight fun in our house!"

Some of your biggest supporters, and best competitors, may be sitting in the next cubicle. If you're someone who's motivated by competition, consider organizing a workplace weight-loss contest. That is, if you can get into a competitive, self-compassionate spirit. Putting your self-loving heart and soul into the competition won't necessarily win you the contest or even stop you from comparing yourself to others, but it will up your odds of finding lasting weight-loss success. And it will ease the fear, self-loathing, and emotional overeating these contests inadvertently inspire.

Despite the many potential pitfalls, workplace contests are popular because the time investment is minimal, and the pay-off is considerable.

Officemates lose on average 12 pounds, about a pound a week, and gain office morale.[17] Besides compassion for yourself and your fellow competitors, the other unspoken challenge that *Biggest Loser*-type contests pose is rebound weight gain. Not to mention motivation, which often gives way to envy and other less admirable feelings after the winner takes all the glory, if not the whole jackpot.

Maybe you would prefer your support with a side of gazpacho or another delicious dish. That's what one of the most creative waist watchers I know, journalist Louisa Kasdon, thought she would try after failing to find an existing group to help her fight the "menopause metabolism-slowing demon" and lose 20 pounds. Why join one more group of strangers in a depressing church basement, she asked herself, when she could invite a team of successful and menopausal career women to get together at a fabulous Cambridge restaurant, where they could weigh in, exchange dieting tips, and share their successes and failures. That one original member owns Upstairs on the Square, one of Harvard Square's finest restaurants, helped launch the club, but didn't ensure its success. In fact, the decadent entrees seemed more likely to inspire weight gain than loss for the members of Down@Up. Which is why the group promptly requested a reduced-calorie menu, and hired an experienced group leader.

"Many of us nursed the fantasy that we'd lose weight automatically just by joining the group," Kasdon later wrote in *More* magazine. "Now we know, there won't be a quick fix. So as we work to become sylphs, we continue to meet for lunch each Wednesday to bolster our vigilance and our sense of humor. We expect to be ladies who lunch

THINK SELF-KIND THOUGHTS

Your Inner Critic:
I hate standing next to skinny people. By comparison, I look like _____ (*fill in the blank*).

Your Compassionate Response:
_____
_____
_____
_____

wisely for a very long time."[18] Lighter ladies. Since the article's publication, many members have happily reached their weight goals. But
while they keep meeting, Kasdon recently reported, they have also
learned that weight-maintenance support is just as important.

Given that obesity plagues pets and pet owners alike, man's best
friend seems like an eager, reliable teammate. (Mind you, unless
you've trained Fluffy to speedwalk, I'm talking about Fido.) At least
he did, until researchers pitted teams of overweight pets and their
pet owners against pet-less waist watchers. Turns out, Fido won't
help you meet any more success than you would romping around
the dog park on your own. But he will make keeping fit more fun and
sociable as he loses three times as much as you do. The enthusiastic
researchers were disheartened to discover that, although the canines
lost 15 percent of their body weight, both sets of human subjects lost
only 5 percent. Actually, the pet-less waist watchers lost a touch more
than the pet owners. Because furry friends are generally ready, willing, and available to go for a walk, researchers remain hopeful that
they will prove themselves as partners in weight maintenance.[19] If you
suspect your dog might be your most encouraging supporter, don't
let one study discourage you. Conduct your own experiment.

Online Support

Face-to-face support groups may sound worthwhile, but if you
can't imagine joining one, or even if you can, online support is
worth considering. Virtual support has distinct advantages and real
disadvantages. On the plus side, it's possible to connect with compassionate community 24–7, instantly, conveniently, and inexpensively,
if not for free. Some time-limited groups limit membership, but the
open-ended majority welcome all comers. In the minus column, not
everyone has Internet access or enough computer savvy to join the
conversation. What's more, online groups can't ensure the same level

of confidentiality that in-person groups can. Nor can they shield members from inaccurate or potentially harmful advice. Most important, virtual weight-loss support is, for the most part, less effective than the real McCoy.[20] But given that the price and accessibility is right, it's the next best thing. To help you navigate the maze of Internet choices, here's an overview of the four main types of support: commercial, academic, professional, and nonprofessional.

Commercial vs. Academic Support

If you're serious about losing weight, you would do better to join an academic e-group than an online commercial program. By academic, I mean any Internet weight-loss program affiliated with a respected university and created by trained professionals. By commercial, I mean self-help sites and other popular diet groups that offer online support in addition to in-person services.

On both commercial and academic sites, you can usually find a group of like-minded waist watchers, a choice of slimming strategies, and various ways to communicate, including message boards. You know, those online bulletin boards without real-life time or space constraints, where members exchange ideas. Academic sites distinguish themselves by offering professionally run weight-management programs, in which students learn cognitive-behavioral concepts in a virtual classroom, recess in chat rooms, and do plenty of homework.

These distinctions are proving worthwhile for active participants. In a study comparing these two types of e-support, subjects who went the academic route not only lost considerably more than those who went commercial, they maintained twice the weight loss, an amount comparable to members of in-person groups. The professional, individualized guidance, researchers believe, makes all the difference, helping academic site-goers get and stay with the program. Those who logged in most, it's worth noting, lost the most.[21]

Nonprofessional Support

Lonely and discouraged dieters desperately seeking hope, under-standing, and diet tips often seek support on websites developed by dieters who were equally lonely and discouraged before they designed winning websites. The sites' catchy mottos provide a glimpse of the dieters you will meet in their chat rooms and on mes-sage boards. If you think "dieting sucks, but bitching about it is fun," for example, you might want to visit a virtual world of disgruntled but determined dieters, and join the bitching party. But if "tips and tricks for hungry chicks" sounds more like your idea of fun, you've got a happy choice of diet sites for cheerier chicks.

Besides providing a forum for girl talk, these sites usually dish up "lite" recipes, "expert" advice, and product reviews. Be forewarned: the web hostess with the mostest may sound like your BFF, but she may be tighter with industry insiders than her friendly subscribers. If you're in the market for this type of peer e-support, do shop around. Some sites are definitely more compassionate and less capitalistic than others.

For a more forgiving perspective, consider subscribing to an online journal, better known as a blog, that takes a kinder view of the human body. To be more specific, think about following a blogger on body image, who challenges the idea that happiness can be measured by the size of your jeans. Body-image bloggers are an impassioned and diverse bunch. They range from outspoken coun-selors, who have watched their eating-disordered clients wither and die before their eyes, to concerned mothers, who are doing all they can to be more self-compassionate role models than their own mothers. These e-journals attract a more loving, accepting crowd than run-of-the-mill diet sites. As do healthy-recipe blogs that fea-ture tasty, whole-food dishes.

PERSONAL SLIMMING LESSON

Chew Gum, Lose Weight?

If you feel like sinking your teeth into something juicy, but are trying to lose weight, food-science researchers suggest you chew gum. In the lab, chewing gum before snack time has been shown to reduce hunger, diminish cravings, promote fullness, and save snackers 25–50 calories. The rationale behind the strategy: small caloric reductions add up to big weight loss.

True enough, but what if you're starving come snack-time? What if your blood sugar's crashing and you need to eat ASAP? What if you can't stomach one more piece of Trident Crystal Frost Fresh Mint gum? Rather than heed the researchers' advice, consider conducting your own experiment. For a day, a week, a month, chew a stick of gum before you break out the cheese and crackers. See if it helps. Before you jump to conclusions, consider your jaw's reaction to routine gum-snapping.

If you're a gambler, consider investing some amount of time and money in one of the diet-betting sites. These websites don't exactly offer positive support, but they do provide community and a forum for competing against friends, family members, co-workers, or oneself. That there's a price to pay—to competitors, a charity, or an anti-charity (one that offends your sensibilities)—has been shown to be a real incentive, especially to overweight men who are generally more comfortable watching team sports than teaming up to watch their waistlines.[22]

From a self-compassionate viewpoint, I'm not convinced that the glee of sticking it to a competitor, the threat of contributing to your least favorite charity, or the humiliation of falling short of your goal, is all that healthy. But the testimonials suggest otherwise. Writes one bettor who describes his pre-betting self as "pudgy and lethargic": "The combination of peer surveillance and the threat of losing money to the Christian right was the perfect combination. I lost 16 pounds, and went from toiling on a treadmill to taking private Pilates lessons . . . all since joining." One can only hope he also gained an ounce of self-compassion.

Ultimately, it's not whether you win or lose, it's how you maintain your weight. After winners and losers are declared, competitors are left with the question that got them betting to begin with: Who you gonna call for support? You can place another bet, of course, or you could form a more cooperative, sustainable partnership.

Professional Support

For more accurate, cutting-edge weight-loss advice, you can trust in the websites hosted by national obesity organizations and other professional groups invested in America's health and well-being. I'm talking about interactive, online communities and other healthy living e-forums created by America's best and brightest, including former U.S. Surgeon General C. Everett Koop, aerobic-exercise forefather Kenneth Cooper, and diet and exercise researcher Miriam Nelson.

Whatever your interest, professional websites are brimming with practical information and expert advice, as well as some, if not all, of the following: assessment tools, newsletters, reading lists, research articles, social networking, and audio and video recordings. If obesity is your main concern, for example, you've got your pick of websites, thanks to organizations like the American Dietetic Association, the American Obesity Association, and the North American Association for the Study of Obesity. If mindfulness is your primary interest, well, there are plenty of websites for that, too. While some professional sites cater to a professional audience, most have much to offer waist watchers with a more personal agenda.

Bottom line: whether you're interested in taking the traditional diet-and-exercise route to losing weight or a more mindful weight-loss approach, you've got many good, reliable choices. For more specific information about the the range of weight-loss supports, be sure to visit Further Reading and Resources.

Whether or not you're any keener on community than you were on the first page of this chapter, by now it should be as clear as bubble wrap that there's something for everyone. That between the mind-blowing choice of actual and virtual groups, there are people somewhere who can do more than encourage you. They can help rewrite your old weight-loss script until it reads: girl meets group, group meets needs, girl succeeds beyond her wildest dreams.

Before you proceed to the next chapter and the practices that will help you find those people, let me leave you with a rhetorical question, this chapter's main point: Why wrestle alone when you can lose significantly more weight, and maybe have more fun, with a winning team?

COMMUNITY-BUILDING
SUGGESTIONS FOR
SEEKING SUPPORT

*It is a fair, even-handed, noble adjustment of things, that while
there is infection in disease and sorrow, there is nothing in the
world so irresistibly contagious as laughter and good-humour.*

CHARLES DICKENS

Weight-loss support. What exactly do you need to succeed? That is the question you will find yourself answering with greater clarity and specificity as you progress through this chapter. For starters, you will actually answer ten questions to gain a general idea of your current support network. After that, as well as a careful review of the individuals and groups who have helped and hindered your progress to date, you will step into the future and the final practice of this chapter with a clear and detailed picture of your winning team.

If you have sampled practices from previous chapters, you will have a good idea what to expect from this one. After the quiz, you will find three writing exercises on weight-loss teams past, present, and future, plus two guided visualizations of social support, for better and for worse. Expect the unexpected in the ultimate practice, the field trip. Rest assured, your field trip will be nothing like the ones your grade-school teachers organized. This time, you're in charge. You get to decide where and when to go.

Q Support sounds good in theory. But, in practice . . . , well, let's just say I've had some bad group experiences. Should I force myself to join up if I'm not up for joining?

A No, forcing yourself is a losing proposition. If you're not ready to seek support, consider getting ready. Your readiness to ask for help, eat more mindfully—to take any positive action—has a lot to do with past experience. Present stage of change, too.

If you're unfamiliar with the Stages of Change model, created by University of Rhode Island psychologist James Prochaska and colleagues,[1] it's worth familiarizing yourself. In Prochaska's view, dieters whose expectations are best summarized by the Nike motto—"Just do it!"—fail to understand that change is a process. A five-stage process: Pre-contemplation, Contemplation, Preparation, Action, and Maintenance.

Dieters expect to wake up New Year's Day in the Action stage, ready to do today what they couldn't manage yesterday, but they're dreaming. More often than not, dieters greet the New Year with the complete and utter ambivalence of Contemplation. That's the stage where a diet may sound like a good idea, but a five-course dinner sounds better. Less often than more, overweight women open their eyes to the heavy denial of Pre-contemplation or the "what, me worry?" stage. Pre-contemplaters might be worried sick about their relatives' weight-related health risks, but not their own. They've got no plans for changing anything anytime soon, like someone who wakes up in the middle of Preparation. Almost ready for action, waist watchers in Preparation are weighing their options, making plans. Positive support is a good idea in every stage, but in Maintenance, it's a winning proposition and one of the secrets to long-term success. In this fifth and final stage, successful waist watchers shift their attention from losing weight to keeping it off.

If you're not ready to jump into action and join a group, don't fret, but do keep in mind: action takes time. Thought and preparation, too.

With every practice in this book, *when* is an important consideration, but it's particularly important with these. That's because before you are good to go through these half-dozen practices, you have got to be good and ready to explore social supports. In my professional experience, neither "good" nor "ready" describes how most waist watchers feel about team efforts. Better words might be "unenthused," "uninterested," "put off," and "opposed." One of the last things clients want to discuss when they first enlist my help is community support.

Ready or not, you can still take a short quiz for a quick snapshot of your current support network. There's also nothing stopping you from entertaining the usual sidebars—taking a Personal Slimming Lesson, finding Thinspiration, thinking Self-Kind Thoughts. When you *are* good and ready to explore where you've been and where you might like to go for your best possible support, you will find the suggested practices provide plenty of direction. Even if finding compassionate community has yet to make your to-do list, one thing you *can* always do is cultivate self-compassion. This very moment, you can take a deep breath and repeat after me:

May I be safe
May I be healthy
May I be happy
May I be fully at ease

Ready for that quiz? If you are, prepare yourself for Jean's Social Support Quiz. Like the Social Support and Eating Habits Survey it's based on, this quiz assesses the negative and positive qualities of your present-day supports. My mindful adaptation of the measure, developed by psychologist James Sallis and his San Diego State colleagues,[2] may be less scientific, but it's quicker and easier, plus I've added scoring guidelines. If you'd rather take the original survey, I wholeheartedly support you. (You can find information about Sallis's quizzes under "Academic" in "Further Reading and Resources.") Grab a quiz, a pencil, and do your best to answer honestly, however imperfectly.

QUIZ 4
Jean's Social Support Quiz

Take this quiz and find out how well your weight-loss support team is working for you. Then do the practices that follow and discover how to build a better team. After you've made a few improvements, retake the quiz. When you compare the two scores, you will see what a quantifiable difference quality support makes to your slimming efforts.

Now consider how often the ten statements below describe your social circle. Next to each statement, note one of the following: none or doesn't apply (n/d), rarely (r), a few times (f), often (o), very often (vo).

In the last three months, one or more friends, relatives, colleagues, neighbors, acquaintances, or other members of my circle:

_____ 1. Encouraged me to skip the chips or resist another temptation.

_____ 2. Complimented me on making healthy food choices.

_____ 3. Expressed genuine interest in my healthy-eating efforts.

_____ 4. Suggested we share in a nutritious snack or meal.

_____ 5. Asked if I'd fallen into old eating habits and needed help getting back on track.

_____ 6. Insisted on eating junk food in my company, knowing full well I'm trying to clean up my diet.

_____ 7. Discouraged healthy menu choices.

_____ 8. Criticized me for wasting money on fresh, whole foods.

_____ 9. Got aggravated when I insisted on eating a healthy dinner.

_____ 10. Encouraged me to overindulge in an indulgence I'm trying to limit or avoid.

Scoring Sheet

For each statement, give yourself 1 point for each "none/doesn't apply"; 2 for "rarely"; 3 for "a few times"; 4 for "often"; and 5 for "very often." Separately total items 1–5 and 6–10. Keep them separate; do not add them together. Record your totals on the lines below:

Total I (1–5): _____   Total II (6–10): _____

Date: _____ / _____ / _____

Your Scores and What to Make of Them

One quiz, two scores? Correct. Total I is a measure of positive support or encouragement. Total II is an indication of negative support or discouragement.

Let's look at the first total first. While accentuating the positive and eliminating the negative is a fantastic idea, a perfect score (Total I: 25, Total II: 5) is just that—a fantasy. Discouragement is a fact of life, especially if you're an unhappily married waist watcher. That said, a high score on Total I (20–25) means you keep exceptionally supportive company. If your first total is more of a halfway measure (13–19), let it encourage you to find a full measure of support. Less than half (12 and under) is no cause for discouragement. If you're self-motivated and already have healthy eating habits, you can get by with less help. But if you keep trying and failing to achieve a healthy, sustainable weight, you can only do better with quality support.

As for your second total, if you scored high on Total II (20–25), you can certainly make the best of a bad situation. But first, face the facts: your situation is bad. You're up against serious discouragement. If yours is an untenable situation, weight loss will have to wait until it becomes more tenable. If it's not all bad, it's good to know that encouragement has a bigger impact on eating habits than discouragement. With enough positive support, you can push past the negative and move forward on weight loss. Plus, your score isn't etched in stone. You could discourage naysayers from saying "nay," or focus on the positive—find extra encouragement by finding more yay-sayers. A middling score (10–19) suggests you would do better with more positive influences and greater distance from negative ones. If you scored in the single digits (1–9), you haven't eliminated the negative, but if you maintain positive connections, you'll up your odds of long-term success.

The Suggestions

In *A Christmas Carol,* a curmudgeonly Scrooge discovers the error of his penny-pinching ways, thanks to the ghosts of Christmas past, present, and future. If Ebenezer Scrooge's favorite exclamation were "I can't believe I ate the whole thing," not "Bah, humbug!" you can be sure the holiday classic would have played differently. If that penny-pincher were a modern mindless eater, those friendly ghosts would undoubtedly take a different route to the same, hopeful ending. To rediscover the gift of mindful eating, a portly Scrooge might need to see a ravenous Tiny Tim devour a bag of Doritos in the sad company of big-screen TV. In the end of this modern-day remake, the miserable loner would still embrace compassionate community and resolve to change his ways, but he would send the Cratchits organic root vegetables and other wholesome side dishes along with a free-range turkey.

In the same holiday spirit, the suggestions you are about to practice will give you the perspective, hope, and resolve that you need to find or expand your compassionate community. Rather than three ghosts, there are six practices to guide you through slimming supports past and present and into a brighter, lighter future. Exactly what your time travels will reveal is unpredictable, but they will surely deliver more of what you have been cultivating all along: good will for one and all. In a word, compassion.

Culled from client conversations and exercises, the upcoming practices are a mix of written exercises, guided visualizations, and field trips. Before you get down to practicing, take a moment to review the suggestions below for practice preparation. For complete instructions, go back to "How to Use This Book."

Ready: All the practices require time and space. How much time? For the first five practices, you will need about fifteen to twenty minutes. The time required for the sixth, the field trip, is unpredictable. Virtual field trips generally take less time than actual excursions. For the real thing, you actually have to get dressed, leave the house, and get where you're going before the learning adventure can begin.

Set: As for space, you will do best in a quiet place that's relatively distraction-free. Whether you prefer writing by hand or keyboard, the writing exercises are best done sitting at a desk or another flat surface. The visualizations are equally effective if you are sitting or lying down wherever you are most comfortable—in an armchair, on a couch or a mat. Your field-trip destination will determine your assumed body position. It's too soon to tell whether you'll be sitting, standing, doing Downward-Facing Dog, or assuming an entirely different position.

Practice: Generally, follow the directions as written. But if you strongly prefer visualizing over writing or vice versa, feel free to mentally guide yourself through a writing assignment, or take writing inspiration from a guided visualization. Whatever you decide, you will need the same tools as before: paper and a writing instrument for the written exercises, or a generous reader or recording device to guide you through the guided visualizations—unless, of course, you prefer to read through a script several times and mentally guide yourself. If you've got *The Self-Compassion Diet* audio program, it won't make practicing any easier this time. I have yet to record any of the social support practices. As for field trips, tool requirements depend on your destination. (More about field-trip preparation later.)

Unlike previous suggestions that cultivate relaxation and are intended for regular practice, these enhance perspective and are for occasional use only. Try them all once, repeating your favorites whenever you like. Keep taking field trips until you find all the encouragement you need. And keep your completed written exercises handy. In the future, your written work will give you invaluable perspective on your current thinking. If there's a caution, it's to avoid jumping to conclusions. Like Scrooge, you might find it hard to imagine how a whirlwind tour of your weight-loss history could be transformative. Or that social support could make much difference. Bah, humbug! If you're serious about sustainable weight loss, suspend judgment, take a leap of faith, and follow me.

FINDING THINSPIRATION

Catch Sarah's Enthusiasm

Successful waist watchers are an enthusiastic and generous bunch, happy to share the secret of their success, and give credit where credit's due . . . to their enthusiastic supporters. The most enthusiastic, intelligent support to come my way came from a dear friend, writing mentor, and co-author of three bestselling fitness books—the late, great Sarah Wernick. Sarah wasn't always so enthusiastic about keeping fit. Before teaming up with Tufts exercise physiologist Miriam Nelson to write *Strong Women Stay Young,* the sedentary author had only disdain for fitness enthusiasts. "Exercise held no appeal for me," she wrote in a *Woman's Day* article. "When I drove past the local women's gym, whose picture windows overlook the street, I laughed at the joggers bobbing on treadmills like gerbils in a cage." In reading, field-testing, and then writing about Nelson's groundbreaking strength-training program, Sarah's tune changed gradually. Three books later and 100 pounds lighter, she maintained her dramatic weight loss, co-authoring another fitness book, exercising with colleagues, and food shopping with friends.

I wasn't in the market for weight-loss inspiration, but I was open to Sarah's encouragement to explore Boston's ethnic markets for new taste treats and the cheapest produce in town. Even when the cancer that would suck the life from this life force made walking difficult, she shopped for her rooibos tea, Greek yogurt, and other favorite foods with hiking poles and a knapsack.

Support like Sarah's doesn't come along every day, nor does it last forever. But her encouragement lives on in the people she loved, the books she wrote, and this Thinspiration. Mark my words: encouragement comes when you least expect it from the most unexpected sources.

PRACTICE 21
Present Company Included: A Writing Exercise

The journey begins with present company or current sources of support. Keeping the Yuletide spirit a bit longer, the first practice asks you to do something like Santa: make a list and check it twice, noting who's been naughty or discouraging, who's been nice and encouraging. In other words, chart and review all supports, positive and negative, actual and virtual. Remember: positive supports facilitate progress; negative ones deter it. Actual support involves people helping people in individual or group therapy, self-help or support groups. Virtual support happens with the help of modern-day technology—on commercial and nonprofit websites, in Internet classrooms, chat rooms, and other e-meeting places.

The simple charts below simplify the writing assignment. Show and tell, actually tell and show, will make the task even simpler. I will tell you about each column, then show you an example.

PRESENT SUPPORT: POSITIVE
Date:

Name	The Thing(s) They Do	Net Effect	Thumbs

PRESENT SUPPORT: NEGATIVE

Date:

Name	The Thing(s) They Do	Net Effect	Thumbs

First, let me tell you about the columns: Under Name, record the names of significant weight-loss supports. List positive supports on the first chart, negative ones on the second. In The Thing(s) They Do column, describe the kinds of things supporters say or do that encourage or discourage your best efforts. Positive supporters, if you remember, do things like express genuine curiosity, give thoughtful compliments and share slimming strategies. Negative supporters are more apt to offer unhealthy snacks, biting criticism, and convincing arguments to skip therapy. Under Net Effect, describe how the things they do generally affect you. In the Thumbs column, use the universal movie critic symbols—one or two thumbs up or down—to rate the impact of each supporter's encouragement or discouragement.

Once you have filled in the blank columns, take a good, close look. What do your yay-sayers have in common? How do your naysayers convey nay? Is there a consistent rhyme to their reason, or any other discernible pattern? Does anyone stand out as exceptionally encouraging or discouraging? Pause, observe, and note your observations on the back of one or both charts.

Now, let me show you my example:

PRESENT SUPPORT: POSITIVE
Date: 1/2010

Name	The Thing(s) They Do	Net Effect	Thumbs
Husband	Helps plan / prepare healthy dinners E-mails articles on nutrition research	Helps make eating healthfully fun & easy	👍👍
Friend Alice	Cooks nutritious, delicious dinners Discusses mindful eating	Inspires my own creative cooking	👍👍
Sister	Shares favorite recipes	Encourages me to try new dishes / foods	👍
Mindfulness Conferences	Lectures by leading experts	Keeps me current Inspires regular meditation practice	👍👍
Harvard Behavioral Medicine Seminar	Presentations on nutrition, mindfulness, self-compassion, and other cutting-edge topics	Keeps me current, excited about my work	👍👍
Yoga Class	Mindfulness meditation in motion	Inspires mindful eating / living	👍

PRESENT SUPPORT: NEGATIVE
Date: 1/2010

Name	The Thing(s) They Do	Net Effect	Thumbs
Husband	Eats snack food in my company	I eat more junk food	👎
Friend JT	Encourages me to drink and be merry	I drink more in his company	👎👎
Aunts	Tell me I should eat more	Feel like they don't understand me	👎
Cousins	Eat only certain carbs	Menu planning can be challenging	👎

Observations

1. I've got more positive support than negative.
2. I'm surprised I don't have MORE positive support, but it seems I've got all I need to eat healthfully and maintain a healthy weight.
3. I'm blessed with a family that enjoys nutritious, delicious meals.
4. While negative support inspires me to eat more mindlessly on occasion, it does me no discernible harm. Plus, chips and salsa, and other less than healthy snacks, are simple pleasures I truly relish.

PRACTICE 22
A Blast from the Past: A Writing Exercise

While my clients need to live, breathe, and eat in the present moment, they also need to learn from the past. I invite them to remember who contributed to their best and worst weight-loss efforts, and on occasion blast back to the imagined past and revisit important influences. This second writing exercise invites you to do much the same. Refocus on then and there. Remember those individuals and groups who helped or hindered weight loss a year or more ago.

The charts for this exercise look like carbon copies of the first. But take a closer look, and you will see they're ever so slightly different:

PAST SUPPORT: POSITIVE
Date:

Name	The Thing(s) They Did	Net Effect	Thumbs

PAST SUPPORT: NEGATIVE
Date:

Name	The Thing(s) They Did	Net Effect	Thumbs

To help you get started, consider the sources of encouragement and discouragement that clients commonly cite. On the discouraging side, clients usually mention one or more of the following: controlling mothers, bullying brothers, naturally slender sisters, and judgmental group leaders. On the encouraging side, it's remarkable how often the most influential individual is cast in both a positive and negative light. A diet group leader, for example, might have been a fountain of encouragement when telling her personal story, but the embodiment of discouragement when talking to members about their weight gain. The most encouraging sources are just as likely to be wholeheartedly positive, and the total opposite of the most discouraging ones. Usual sources of all-positive support include energetic aerobics instructors, empathic psychotherapists, celebrity waist watchers, like-minded family members, and beloved dogs.

If you did the first writing practice, review your present-day charts after charting past supports, but before drawing any conclusions. Even if you didn't do the previous practice, take a moment to look for patterns. Notice what's changed, and what's remained the same. Did you have more or less support in earlier weight-loss efforts? If you have fewer supports in the present, are there past connections you would consider remaking or replicating? If you have more or markedly different support, are all current supports worth maintaining? Pause, reflect, and record your reflections on the chart's flip side.

Got it? Get ready. Go!

PRACTICE 23
In Good Company: A Guided Visualization

All waist watchers need encouragement, even the happy successes. The happiest may not need more encouragement, but none are immune to discouragement. And none are more easily or quickly discouraged than the least successful waist watchers. Rather than risk another discouraging word, interaction, or situation, the least likely to succeed turn their backs on their slimming plans and open their mouths for comfort food. Until, that is, they gain another five or ten pounds and—well, you know how that vicious cycle goes.

If you're interested in getting off that lonely, broken-down merry-go-round and climbing aboard a more sociable, workable one, you will want to try this guided visualization. It's really three visualizations in one: (1) a reunion with encouragement, (2) a second chance with discouragement, and (3) a date with success. If you are short on time, feel free to do one part and try the others later. Any part you find particularly challenging, keep practicing it over time until you've mastered it. Even if you've got plenty of positive support and next to no negative, you won't want to miss the perspective and inspiration all parts provide in toto.

Visualization 1

Take a moment to make yourself comfortable, let go of the day's concerns, and allow the breath to settle into a quiet, steady rhythm. Without force or effort, simply invite the inhalation to deepen, the

PERSONAL SLIMMING LESSON

Ban Supernormal Stimuli?

According to psychologist Deirdre Barrett, a Harvard Medical School colleague, America's junk food addiction can be explained in one term: supernormal stimuli. "Super-cali-what?" Nope, "supernormal stimuli," a term Barrett borrows from the study of animal behavior to describe supersweet, fatty, or otherwise unnaturally appealing food.

"We're programmed to forage for sugar and saturated fats because these were once found only in hard to come by fruit and game," she writes in her 2007 book *Waistland: The (R)Evolutionary Science Behind Our Weight and Fitness Crisis*. "Now this programming lures us powerfully toward plastic-wrapped hunks of corn syrup solids and hydrogenated vegetable oils."[3] Super-appealing snacks and meals, the scholarly psychologist believes, trigger changes in the same brain chemicals affected by heroin and other addictive drugs.

Barrett's antidote to the obesity epidemic may have been considered radical before *Waistland*'s publication, but since then, several best-selling authors have prescribed the same spartan diet. If you've ever tried to eat just one potato chip and wound up eating the whole bag, swearing off chips could prove a worthwhile experiment.

But should you ban all supernormal stimuli forever? That's not my choice, but if it were, I would start with a mini-ban. Before resigning myself to a lifetime of berries and nuts, I would try eating like a cavewoman for a week or two.

exhalation to lengthen. When you're ready, imagine a school, community center, or some other public place with a never-ending corridor and an infinite number of doors. In your mind's eye, look around. See what it's like to be in a place dedicated to positive support. Gazing down this endlessly long hall of doors, it's only natural to wonder what you'll discover in this vast supportive place.

Your first discovery is that there's little time for wondering. The echo of your first tentative steps suddenly transports you to a door . . . a door to a time and place where you felt your best: calm, clear, capable, and most of all, supported. Crack the door, peek inside. If the room doesn't contain good memories of positive supports, try another, until you find a room full of encouragement.

Let yourself in and let your senses bring the scene to life. See, feel, and hear what it's like to be greeted by warm smiles—to join compassionate company, to welcome positive support. Go ahead, see where you are, what's going on, who's here. You'd recognize those faces anywhere, and yet you'd forgotten how much you've missed their companionship. How their very presence makes you feel both comforted and energized. As you remember and maybe even reexperience what it's like to feel fully accepted, if not unconditionally loved, you breathe a sigh of relief. With every in-breath, you feel a deeper sense of comfort and ease. With every out-breath, greater energy and health. Feeling ease on the inhale, health on the exhale. Whenever you could use some positive energy, simply and silently repeating "ease" as you inhale, "health" as you exhale.

Like a mantra: Ease . . . Health . . . Ease . . . Health . . .

Visualization 2

These feelings of health and ease will stay with you as you say good-bye to this supportive group, and head next door to a time and place when you felt discouraged about weight loss. In this next room, you won't find your most discouraging memory, but you will find a somewhat disheartening one that involves someone disappointing who did more to discourage than encourage you. A memory you'd be willing to reexperience, so you can relearn how to handle negative support more positively. More effectively. But this time, you'll have help. A compassionate advisor of your choice. A fictional character or a living, breathing, caring person who'll make sure your re-education is a positive one.

Before you walk through that door, reacquaint yourself with the wise soul who's ready to advise and protect you. Happy to help you breathe deeply, conduct yourself differently, deal with old, uncomfortable feelings if they arise. Rest assured, you'll feel no more than you can comfortably handle. Your advisor will see to that.

As soon as you enter this discouraging room, you feel the negativity. The light is dim, the air is heavy, but the negative energy doesn't stop you from looking into the dark corners of your weight-loss history. You can see or remember where you are, who's there, what they're doing, saying, intimating. As the scene starts replaying in your mind's eye, the feelings, sensations, and perceptions start returning. It's happening much the same, but differently. For one thing, with your advisor at your side, you're feeling calmer, wiser, stronger. Feeling as secure as you do, it takes no time to rewrite history. To stare disappointment in the face and see it in perspective. It takes no time at all to refresh a sense of "ease" with the inhale, "health" on the exhale. And do what you couldn't do before—stand up for yourself, speak your mind . . . do whatever it takes to right this wrong and maintain your dignity. Before you close the door on this experience and say goodbye to your advisor, you inhale fully, exhale slowly, and suffuse the room with positive energy.

Visualization 3

Your curiosity propels you into the hall and on to one last room. Behind this door resides your future self at a healthy, sustainable weight. Step right in. She's expecting you. Yes, that's you: attractive, healthy, radiant. What a world of difference mindful weight loss has made to your facial expression, your posture, your waistline. Can you believe you traded in those baggy outfits for more form-fitting fashions? Even if your picture of health is hard to see, or nothing like you imagined, notice what's different—physically, mentally, and emotionally—about a slimmer, more mindful you.

Now, expand your focus to encompass the compassionate company your future self keeps. Note who's there, how they're communicating, what they're doing or offering that's especially helpful. What's most surprising? That you've found positive support? That you rely on it? Or is it that you've achieved a healthy, sustainable weight? That if you regain a pound or two, you don't panic? You know what helps you get back on track, and you trust yourself enough to return to what you know. The biggest surprise isn't the number on the scale, the shape of your body, or the fit of your clothes, is it? No, it's the feeling you get giving and taking. The pleasure of helping and being helped. You had no idea how much you'd enjoy the give-and-take of it all.

Before you close the door on this supportive group, take an imaginary group picture for your mental screen-saver. Whenever you're short on hope or vision, there they'll be. Just a glance away. You can always revisit this supportive atmosphere another time, but right now, it's time to take a deep inhalation, a long, slow exhalation. And bring your attention to present reality, the first moment of your encouraging future.

PRACTICE 24
Worlds Apart: A Guided Visualization

Picturing yourself on a winning weight-loss team is one thing, actively participating is quite another. If you are like most dieters, you have got many good reasons why it's not such a great idea to make weight loss a team effort. Maybe you've been there, done that. Maybe, despite the encouraging news about teamwork, you would still rather do it yourself. If you feel the least bit ambivalent about positive support, this visualization is for you. If you've already found a long-term group you can call your own, congratulations! And enjoy the view this practice affords of where you've been and where you still might like to go.

Settle into a comfortable position and a quiet breathing rhythm, and ready yourself for two must-see videos. But first, in your mind's eye, imagine a computer screen. A large, full-color monitor that's easy to see as you naturally breathe deeply, slowly, and quietly. Topping today's playlist is a video about a lonely dieter. Hit the imaginary play button, and watch someone like you step on the scale with her best intentions. She's every dieter on Monday morning: determined to lose weight once and for all. She's set on being "good." In other words, undereating, overexercising, if not both. Even if she takes an exercise class or confides in a friend about her renewed efforts, she's fighting the battle of the bulge as an army of one.

Her virtuous start is familiar. So is the thrill of stepping on the scale days later, pounds lighter. Getting dressed, she reminds herself that nothing tastes sweeter than weight-loss success, and quickly calculates how many weeks it will take to reach her goal. Somehow she's miscalculated. In a matter of days, her optimism gives way to pessimism. Like a highway wreck, your eyes are drawn to the wreckage. After a series of small, but significant moments—a skipped meal here, an extra cookie there—the pounds she lost start piling back on. She tells herself it's not the end of the world, but with every ounce regained, she sounds less convinced. The day the pounds gained outweigh the pounds lost, you brace yourself for the inevitable.

With no positive support to speak of, the lonely dieter has little protection against thoughtless comments and biting criticisms. Her pain is uncom-

THINK SELF-KIND THOUGHTS
Your Inner Critic:
(*Fill in your harshest criticism about your least favorite body part.*) _____
Your Compassionate Response:
_____
_____
_____
_____

fortably familiar, and you don't want to feel it. You hit fast-forward, and there she is, overwhelmed, more alone than ever. Rather than get swallowed up by distress, you watch her do what you've done—swallow the highest-calorie treats in sight. You can't bear to watch her punish herself another second. And you can't imagine this woeful tale ending happily, and you can't stomach the idea of watching the bitter end. So you stop the action, and proceed to the second video about a globe-trotting waist watcher.

From the first frame, you're breathing more easily. Like that feel-good video about the dorky guy who asks the world to dance, this globe-trotter invites global support. One minute, she's meditating on an orange with a Vietnamese monk; the next she's attending a potluck meal with a peaceable group of Israeli–Palestinian waist watchers. Before you know it, she's signing up for a mindfulness study at a Harvard teaching hospital. Unlike the lonely dieter who postpones living for tomorrow, this gal seizes the day, the experience, the support. Virtually and actually. After a class on an academic weight-loss website, she joins an online chat about slimming contests, and e-mails a friend her favorite mindful-eating video.

The globe-trotter's adventures in interconnection inspire you to imagine your own. To envision your own global village of support. To flip through your mental Rolodex of friends, relatives, colleagues, trainers, therapists . . . anyone and everyone who might like to make weight-loss a common cause. Before you know it, you're entertaining lots of exciting possibilities, and watching the credits roll. Wow! Lost in thought, you got the message, but you missed the video's ending. You'd like to see how it ends. You're definitely interested in the payoff of positive support.

PRACTICE 25
Future Support Now: A Writing Exercise

Who you gonna call for positive support? That is the question you have been entertaining for almost two chapters, and by the end of this practice you'll have a good, working list of personalized answers. Yup, it's that time again—time to make one last chart.

But first, this writing exercise dares you to dream. To entertain all future support possibilities—your wildest dreams (a personal chef, an extended spa vacation), new possibilities (group psychotherapy, a mindful-eating class), and oldies but goodies (a self-help group, a walking club). Dreaming up ideas may sound doable, but when I dare clients to dream about future support, many nix possibilities before they can consider them. If you find yourself dismissing future teammates as soon as you imagine them, notice this nixing impulse and invite your imaginary team to stay a while.

The chart you are about to fill in is not much different than the others, but you are. This time, you are looking ahead. Instead of today or yesterday, you are focused on tomorrow. You will see that the columns look the same, but given your future focus, the directions are a little different. Take a look, then we'll talk directions:

FUTURE SUPPORT
Date:

Name	The Thing(s) They'll Do	Net Effect	Thumbs

Okay, now the directions: In the Name column, list possible sources of *future* support: individuals (friends, relatives, colleagues, therapists, dogs) *and* groups (nonprofit, commercial, therapeutic, academic, your own creation). Forget about listing negative future supports, focus only on the positive. In listing positive supports, be as specific as possible. Instead of "diet group," write the name of the group you're thinking about joining (Weight Watchers, Overeaters Anonymous). If you like the idea of a psychotherapy group, note the kind of group you're considering (mindful-eating group, cognitive-behavioral therapy). That is, if you happen to know it.

For each support, describe what you hope it will give you (encouragement, education, perspective, relaxation . . .) under The Thing(s) They'll Do. In the Net Effect column, record the hoped-for result of getting that support (feel less isolated, more self-accepting). Under Thumbs, rate the promise of each option using the movie critics' rating system (single or double thumbs-up or thumbs-down). Ideally, you'll finish the exercise with a minimum of three solid options. If none of your best options earned two thumbs up, try this exercise again after asking others about their favorite supports.

If you've completed the Past and Present Support charts, reviewing both will jump-start the brainstorming process. Even if you have yet to fill in the blanks on the previous charts, combing through your weight-loss history for your most enthusiastic supporters will help you imagine who will best support your continuing weight-loss efforts. You're generally focusing on positive, not negative supports, but keep in mind that negative supports can be positive influences. Under certain circumstances, some of your biggest naysayers can be your most enthusiastic yay-sayers. Take my husband, for example. Although he encourages me to eat less-than-nutritious snacks on occasion, he's always happy to help cook nutritious, delicious meals. Also, don't forget about successful supporters you have yet to meet or barely know (a therapist who comes highly recommended, a nutritionist you've been meaning to call, an inspiring mindfulness instructor).

Finally, this chart is meant to be a work in progress. After investigating your best options, you will want to make updates, modifications, additions, subtractions. Continue your investigation until you find what you're looking for: your winning team.

PRACTICE 26
Good to Go: A Field Trip

You have traveled a considerable distance over the course of this chapter, and you have come full circle. After visiting support past and future, you are back to the present. Same time zone, different altitude. You now have a higher perspective of the support you need to reach your ultimate destination: a healthy, sustainable weight. Plus, you're in a better position than the average dieter who is desperate to believe diet ads' pie-in-the-sky promises. Desperation not only enhances gullibility, it drastically reduces the odds of meeting your needs. Having a clearer idea of your support needs puts you in a better position, but to find your dream team or strengthen your existing one, you will do best with a detailed picture of the team's players, their track record (if they have one), and winning strategies.

The best way I know to get the necessary details is to take a field trip. As a student, you had no say about trip destinations. You went where and when you were told. Many waist watchers expect as much—to be told what, if not when, to eat. But, as I'm sure you've noticed, I guide with suggestions, not hard-and-fast rules. What follows are my suggested guidelines for your upcoming learning adventure.

Start with One: Begin with your best support option and see where it leads. If you're interested in an established group, look beyond the advertised promises and into consumer reviews and current research. If reliable sources like *Consumer Reports* and Google Scholar (the popular search-engine's database of scholarly articles) can't tell you how your best bet compares with the rest, get an expert opinion from, well, an expert (a trusted health-care provider, respected academic, successful waist watcher). If you are more inclined to create your own group, interview potential members as well as those who have formed similar groups. If your field work reveals your best option is as good, or better, than you expected, don't stop there. Take at least one more trip for comparison.

How many field trips does it take to find a winning team? Only you can decide. But if the first one leaves you feeling less than impressed, keep searching until you find what you're looking for.

Anticipate Questions: To make a wise investment of your time, energy, if not your discretionary cash, you will need simple answers to a basic list of questions: What's the plan? Who's involved? How much does it cost? Where and when do members meet? Your preliminary investigation may reveal much of the factual information you need to assess a group's effectiveness, convenience, and affordability, but it may not give you enough emotional feedback to make an informed choice. Consider how you want to feel as an active participant (safe, comfortable, included, respected?) as well as how you don't want to feel (unwelcomed, ignored, criticized). Once you've got a question list in mind—or better yet, in hand—you're almost good to go.

Bring a Friend?: Waist watchers can increase their comfort by turning field trips into group shopping expeditions. Why not take comfort in numbers? If you've got a like-minded friend who's good to go on a field trip, great! She just might be your most enthusiastic supporter. But she could just as easily be a good excuse to set aside your needs and take care of hers. Before you make your field trip a group project, question your motives and hers. If you really think a friend or two will enrich your learning adventure, by all means, bring 'em along. But if you suspect you've got mixed motives or they've got conflicting agendas, travel solo.

Make a Date: Before you schedule a field trip, keep in mind that learning whatever you need to learn takes time. How much time largely depends on your destination. Virtual trips can be quicker if you've got Internet access and enough computer savvy. After all, you can travel the World Wide Web without stepping out of your pajamas or the front door. If your computer access and support lives elsewhere, virtual travel takes longer. If you're crazy busy, you can always take several short online trips instead of one long one.

By far, actual field trips take the longest and the most planning. Some groups are open to all comers; others welcome newcomers by appointment only. If you're lucky, you will get a choice of introductory meetings. If not, you've got no choice but to meet where and when members meet. Unless, of course, you decide to create your own support group. Bottom line: wherever you go, give yourself enough time to check out the plan and the participants.

Cultivate Self-Compassion: If you're underwhelmed by the prospect of a field trip, you've got plenty of company and, no doubt, a good reason or three. Rather than try to kick yourself into gear, consider practicing loving-kindness. Accept the fact that as much as you may want or need support, you're not quite ready for it. Kindly remind yourself that action follows thought and planning, if not some amount of hopelessness, dissatisfaction, doubt, fear, impatience, hope, and vision.

If you're not prepared for a formal excursion, it doesn't mean you're unprepared for an informal study. It takes virtually no effort to listen to what successful waist watchers are saying about positive support. Or to notice if an article you're reading about a weight-loss group piques your interest. You will seek support when you're good and ready. Until then, a little self-compassion goes a long way.

Practice Patience: To go along with self-compassion, your learning adventure will go better with a little patience. Unless you live in a distant, TV-free galaxy, there's enormous pressure to lose weight. Whatever the source—your significant other, primary-care physician, yourself—it's easy to buckle under the unbearable heaviness of our thin-crazed culture, and join the club that promises the fastest results. Pressured decisions and impulse purchases can pay off in the short run, but long-term they backfire big-time. If patience isn't one of your virtues, catch some. Hang out with an extra-patient personal or professional relation. Like healthy eating habits, patience is positively contagious. Besides resisting pressure, patience comes in handy if you have to take more field trips than expected, or make several visits to the same group in a different locale. It's especially handy if your desired support turns out to be less than desirable. Like food shopping when you're starving, seeking support when you're impatient can be costly.

PART V

Continuing Education

*The Power of
Personal Persistence*

ULTIMATE SUGGESTIONS FOR FILLING YOUR TOOLBOX

I was drowning and she [Julia Child] pulled me out of the ocean.

JULIE POWELL

I love a good list. Not the same way I love a good home-cooked meal, but I find lists clarifying, motivating, and ultimately satisfying when all to-dos are done and deleted. I could wax on about list-making, but isn't this chapter about filling your toolbox? Exactly, and shortly, without formality, you will understand why lists and tools go hand in hand.

Chapter 9 won't ask you to fill out formal to-do lists to figure out what *to do* with your new set of weight-loss tools. It will, however, offer a few simple suggestions for sorting through the tools you've acquired over the course of this book and your dieting lifetime, and building a better, more personalized toolbox. For the most part, the ninth chapter will give you time, space, and experience to reflect on where you've been and where you are now. With a better appreciation of all you have learned, you can take one last Personal Slimming Lesson and entertain the other usual sidebars, then proceed to the afterword, where you'll find an early acquaintance from the preface: the impatient dieter.

Now to get back to the original question: how do lists and tools go hand in hand? Lists help you build a better toolbox. A good, short list also helps you heed the best piece of personal advice from early American writer Henry David Thoreau: "Simplify, simplify." Of course, when the mindful author penned that pithy quote from his cabin with a view, he was writing about living life deliberately, not losing weight mindfully. Since I am typing a stone's throw from his Walden Pond writing retreat and the desks of other great authors, Concord's rich literary tradition moves me to share some mindful deliberations of my own on the topic at hand.

To build your best possible toolbox, constructing a favorite tool list is the simplest, easiest thing you can do. Make one long list of favorite practices, favorite groups, favorite books, and other favorite resources that have previously proven helpful. Taking note of the real keepers—the ones that changed your eating for the better, at least for a while—gives you a real chance of finding what you need when you really need it. If you do better with lists that are shorter than longer, here's a helpful hint: write several short ones. Of course, if you're not into list-making, find your best way to get organized. But if you're into little lists, consider making one or more of the following:

1. Most Promising Practices is a list of your favorite practices from *The Self-Compassion Diet.* Of the twenty-six-plus practices contained in these pages and listed on pages ix–x, make a short list of the chosen few that are worth repeating, if not working into your routine. Adding a favorite practice to this short list isn't the same thing as making a lifetime commitment. If there's a favorite one you would like to practice regularly, go for it. Otherwise, keep your options open. Entertain a variety.

2. Leading Support Options is what it sounds like—your best options for weight-loss support. Of the various kinds of in-person and

PERSONAL SLIMMING LESSON

Retrain Your Taste Buds?

Taste buds are incredibly adaptable. Eat a steady diet of almost anything, and you'll likely acquire a taste for it. Some nutritionists take this simple fact to mean lasting weight loss requires systematic taste-bud retraining. To their way of thinking, following set menus, if not specific recipes, is a waist watcher's only hope of taking pleasure in foods that pack the most nourishment in the fewest calories.

Mindful-eating experts have more natural ways of helping dieters develop a taste for a healthy diet. One of the simplest, most intuitive practices comes from Lillian and Leonard Pearson's groundbreaking book, *The Psychologist's Eat Anything Diet*.[1] While the Pearsons never described their practice as a taste-bud retraining strategy, it certainly and effectively is. Here's the idea: dieters naturally desire nutritious, delicious food when they subsist on a diet consisting of mostly "humming foods" and occasionally "beckoning foods."

What's the difference? A humming food is what you know you want to eat before you see, smell, or taste it. It's the answer to the question: What would really hit the spot? Something sweet or salty, smooth or crunchy, hot or cold? When you crave a humming food, only a specific taste, texture, and temperature will do. If you crave a warm chocolate-chip cookie, for example, an icy carrot stick won't cut it. Or if you're humming for a bowl of bran cereal, eggs Benedict holds no appeal. Humming foods aren't always readily available, but they're usually worth the wait because they satisfy physical and emotional hunger.

Conversely, beckoning foods are convenient and plentiful. The main reason diners order such a food is the same one mountain climbers cite: because it's there. Take birthday cake, for example. Partygoers usually do. Doesn't matter if they're stuffed or the frosting is sickly sweet: if everyone's having cake, they're eating it, too. Beckoning foods call to your senses . . . when you see them rolling on dessert carts, smell them wafting from the pizza oven, hear them blending in the Frappuccino maker. Because what beckons is typically tasty but ultimately unsatisfying, if you indulge you risk overindulging.

In short, satisfy a hum, end of craving. Get enticed by a beckon, and don't be surprised if it leaves you feeling unsatisfied, if not insatiable. At least that's the theory. But is the dietary practice of satisfying hums for you? Try it, see if you like it.

online support described in chapter 7, which ones pique your interest, give you hope? Whatever your interest—professional or nonprofessional, commercial or academic, individual or group therapy, create your own or join the diet club—shortlist any and all team efforts you would consider (re)joining or creating. Be as specific as you can with names of potential organizations, websites, therapists, and so on.

If you've already got good support, take an example from Mark and Alex, the guys who halved their body weight with Overeaters Anonymous. Stick with a good thing. Last time they e-mailed, Mark was happily maintaining his 155-pound weight loss, which is no small task given that he's the proud daddy and primary caretaker of a baby boy. Alex had slipped back into old eating habits for a while, but he never gave up. "I managed to put back about 20 pounds [of the 160 he had lost]," he wrote, "but have lost about half of it in the past month. It's certainly harder maintaining than losing the weight, but by working the program, there's no way I'll let the weight creep back."

3. Best Tools Ever is a list of those favorite few that have really come in handy over the years. Literally handy. Trusty tools you've held in your hands or that required the use of your hands, like healthy cookbooks, mindful-eating CDs, exercise videos—real things that rescued you from despair, and helped you eat as you've always wanted to eat. Like Julia Child's *Mastering the Art of French Cooking* saved Julie Powell, the author of *Julie & Julia*. Except, unlike Julia's cookbook, your lifesaving thing(s) have helped you indulge more in delicious, nutritious recipes, and less in super-rich cuisine.

THINK SELF-KIND THOUGHTS

Your Inner Critic:

_____ (*Fill in your meanest thoughts about your eating.*)

Your Compassionate Response:

_____

_____

_____

_____

4. Future Wish List is a short note to yourself about tools you might like to add to your personal collection in the future. It's an ongoing to-do list of intriguing practices, books, groups, healthy vacations, and other things you don't have to do, but might really enjoy doing. Because it's a wish list, anything goes on it: a mindful-living community in the French countryside, a working vacation on an organic farm, cooking lessons in a Zen kitchen. If you like the idea of meditating in a cave with a view, visiting an Indian ashram, consulting a Balinese medicine man, don't let practicality get in the way. By committing pen to paper, you're making no firm commitments. You're simply entertaining possibilities.

You could continue entertaining future possibilities or turn your attention to more pressing matters—summarizing lessons learned, underscoring key points and doing other book-ending ceremonies.

Yes, I'm asking you to mindfully focus your awareness on your breath, something I've been asking

NO STUPID QUESTIONS

Q All my friends swear by cleansing diets, but I'm not sure ridding my body of toxins will help me lose weight. What do you think?

A I'm not a big fan of cleanses. I don't think human toxins build up like so much gunk on oven walls. Nor do I think liquid or solid-food cleanses can cure obesity or right other long-standing nutritional wrongs.

That said, when mindfully followed, cleansing has proven illuminating, if not curative, for at least one client. Despite my discouraging words, this client was convinced a two-week cleanse would help her lose a few pounds, if not ease her chronic stomach pain. To my amazement and her delight, not only did she lose weight, but her digestive distress decreased, enabling her doctor to diagnose a previously undiagnosed condition.

Personal experience can be persuasive, and yet there's no scientific evidence to suggest cleansing is a sustainable weight-loss strategy. Personally I've never done a cleanse, but I did try a yummy-sounding cauliflower-and-carrot soup recipe from a cleanse-enthusiast's cookbook. When my taste buds asked for more, I happily ladled myself a second and third bowl. If only I had read the fine print. Enough said.

you to do directly and indirectly from the beginning. By now, I expect you know the mindful-breathing drill. Make yourself comfortable, focus on the most vital aspect of your breathing (the rise and fall of your chest, the air at the entrance of your nostrils), and when the mind naturally wanders, refocus on breathing. But are you aware that awareness is more than a drill? It's the handiest tool in the toolbox.

AWARENESS: THE ALL-PURPOSE TOOL

For nearly nine chapters, *The Self-Compassion Diet* has given you a good deal of certainty—current research, proven practices, and other tried-and-true slimming strategies. But at times on your weight-loss journey, you will feel more and less sure of yourself. At some point, you are bound to meet terrifying uncertainty. I'm not trying to scare you, but just prepare you for those inevitable moments when you feel ill-equipped. If your toolbox is handy in such a moment, great! Open the latch, grab a familiar tool. If your toolbox is unavailable, or your tools suddenly unfamiliar, no need to panic. There's one all-purpose tool you can always use. Need a hint? It's an integral part of self-compassion. It's awareness.

If you only remember one thing, remember this: the more you carefully hone your awareness, the more you gently train your attention on your own experience, the more you kindly observe your reactions and interactions, the more you can honestly trust that you've got what you need to succeed. To appreciate the great, enduring value of awareness, you can always review the mindfulness chapters. But I have two lasting reminders on mindful awareness. You'll get the first reminder through firsthand experience. You'll get the second one through secondhand experience. It's a story.

First, the firsthand experience. Bring your awareness to the book you are holding in your hands. Notice the size and weight of the book, the number of remaining pages. Whether it's an old-fashioned book or a newfangled electronic device, remember the hopes you held in the first chapter. Consider the distance you've come in nine chapters. Consider all you've learned. On some level, you're aware of the approaching crossroads. It's the intersection of endings and beginnings. If you're in the habit of rushing to new beginnings, it's easy to miss this important junction. But stay focused on your experiencee, and you'll see that it's a worthwhile resting place.

Now that you're here, permit yourself to pause, breathe, rest. To experience whatever you experience. To notice whatever you notice from a self-compassionate viewpoint. It's hard not to notice that soon we'll part ways. You'll go your way, and I'll go mine. Partings, perhaps you've noticed, can inspire mixed feelings and shallow breathing. If you're breathing more from the chest, less from the belly, kindly deepen your inhalation, carefully lengthen your exhalation. As you deepen your breathing, shift your awareness to feelings. Just noticing the mix of feelings, but changing nothing. Awareness changes nothing and everything. The facts don't change: our paths are still diverging, and you remain concerned about your eating habits. The next leg of your journey is still to come.

But perceptions do shift and change. Practicing awareness, as you are right now, you're not just breathing, you're appreciating the fresh inspiration of each in-breath, the calming influence of each out-breath. Practicing awareness, the next leg of the journey is this moment. The destination isn't someplace better; there's no better place to be than right here. Practicing awareness is breathing and appreciating: There's no place like here. There's no place like here. There's no place like here.

Keep breathing and prepare yourself for the second reminder. Yes, it's story time. So sit back, make yourself comfortable again, and I'll tell you the story of a bulimic client of mine. Like many waist watchers, this dedicated dieter had a box full of weight-loss tools she rarely used, and a few reliable diet tricks up her sleeve. For four decades, this fortysomething interior designer kept a handle on her food and her mood by starving, binging, and occasionally purging. Until, that is, a bad breakup forced her to face three awful truths: she had lost the love of her life, put on 15 pounds, and her reliable diet tricks had stopped doing the trick.

Despair sent her packing and soul-searching on Martha's Vineyard, the funky island off the Cape Cod coast. There she spent long days exploring empty beaches under panoramic skies, farmstands over-flowing with fresh produce, glorious sunsets casting light upon fishing

FINDING THINSPIRATION

Hope Springs Eternal

Winter's tough on weight-loss inspiration. A cool, gray day mid-fall or spring can be refreshing, but a full season of inclement weather can be downright depressing. Winter drives dieters inside and away from important supports. Even those who enjoy winter sports and a strong support network find gray skies, chilly temperatures, and inferior produce more than a little discouraging. Unless you live in the tropics or go south with the snowbirds, there's no escaping the fact that frigid air encourages the rest of us to hunker down to heartier meals, if not a more sedentary lifestyle.

If only northern waist watchers could remember that winter weight gain is like a fleece jacket—it's natural to put it on by Christmas and take it off well before Memorial Day. Sadly, most tend to forget that cravings for lean cuisine and physical activity return with the robins, that interest in weight loss resurfaces with the crocuses. I can prompt clients to remember this seasonal truth, but prompting, however reassuring, can't resurrect hope.

Happily, hope's usually right around the corner, if not closer. If you're low on Thinspiration, you need look no further than your backyard garden, if you have one. Or any place hope springs eternal: flower shops, community gardens, local farms, farmer's markets. If you live in a concrete jungle, look for hope in public gardens, window boxes, and produce markets. But if you can't find Thinspiration anywhere, you can always order it—at least in California, where franchises deliver organic vegetable gardens and vineyards direct to your doorstep.

villages. She had planned on spending evenings in quiet introspection, but instead she found herself in hearty dinner conversation with her new island friends. Breathing, eating, and living like an islander, she was surprised how much calmer, happier, and healthier she felt.

Even more surprising was her sudden lack of interest in her old diet tricks, and new interest in a handy, yet unfamiliar tool: awareness. The slow island pace and fresh local cuisine made it easy to practice what had seemed nearly impossible back home: To eat mindfully. To enjoy satisfying portions of delicious, nutritious food. Without starving, binging, or purging, mindfully attending to her mood proved more difficult than food. But with a little help from this friendly community, she's a little better at dealing with feelings that used to trigger binges. She's also more than a little curious about what the bathroom scale will say about her mindful weight-loss approach over time now that she's naturally lost the 15 pounds she had gained.

This story is unfolding, but this book is coming to a close. So let's cut to the moral: pause, breathe, rest, open yourself to experience, revel in nature, befriend mixed feelings, enjoy seasonal cuisine and hearty conversation, keep good, supportive company. But most of all, kindly pay attention. The more you pay attention to your unfolding journey, the more you see there's only one way to go. Your way. It might not be the most direct route, but it's heading in the right direction. Even with the best GPS or the most careful itinerary, there's no sure way to anticipate wrong turns and dead ends. But if you forge ahead with open eyes and a kind heart, rest assured that you will find your way.

Before you go on your way, it's worth circling back to the beginning. Like before-and-after photos, see how the dieter behind *The Self-Compassion Diet* is doing. She would love to say a quick hello and a proper good-bye. If you drop by the afterword, the next little chapter, you'll find her there.

AFTERWORD

The Compassionate Guide

Life itself is the proper binge.
JULIA CHILD

There you are, looking more relaxed and self-compassionate than the day we met. A little more mindful, too. I'm glad you could drop in before setting out on the next leg of your journey. You've come quite a distance, haven't you? So have I. When I first started my weight-loss journey three-plus decades ago, I was afraid I wouldn't get very far. My mom's dieting girlfriends gave me good reason to fear that I, too, would always be an impatient dieter. Even after I graduated to figure-salon manager, syndicated fitness columnist, and psychotherapy grad student, I never believed I would ever get where I was going.

As I reach the end of *The Self-Compassion Diet,* I can clearly see how far I have come in thirty-odd years. Here I am, a mindful eater and compassionate weight loss guide, fully appreciating that right here is the best possible place to be.

When I first proposed this book, I expected the writing to be challenging. But I had good reason to believe I would fare healthier than colleagues who had suffered weight gain, migraines, and marital difficulties in the book-writing process. For one: because I had learned to maintain my weight long ago, I didn't expect to gain weight, and I didn't. Second: I had an added advantage—a remarkably supportive husband.

My mind and body met the challenge, but they did pay the price. Sitting and typing day after day is more fatiguing than any exercise regimen, and time-consuming, leaving me less time to work out than I like. I made time to nourish my body, but I deprived my taste buds of delightful variety. When they couldn't take one more quick-and-easy dinner, I took them out to eat or got take-out. My mind's still sharp, but it's hard to recall when my attention span was long enough to enjoy playing Scrabble. I imagine it was well before my meditation practice fell off the cushion and crawled into bed.

Book-writing has been demanding, but it's also been illuminating and transformative. Researching the psychological routes to sustainable weight loss has changed the way I work. I now spend more time listening, understanding, and offering support, and less time scrutinizing, analyzing, and advising. My research has also changed the way I close cases. It's no longer enough to wrap up treatment by summarizing weight-maintenance strategies. Even when happy clients say they're good to go, our work isn't finished until they have entertained possibilities for ongoing support.

Speaking of support, besides daily contact with my husband, I have met weekly with Harvard Medical School colleagues, but I have seen far less of everyone else. Online social networking is a marvelous innovation, but it's no substitute for in-person interactions.

As I close the book on this book, my first order of business is people, shutting off Facebook and catching up with friends and family face-to-face. Mind and body are the second and third orders of business. My mind craves calming activities, like sitting on the beach or floating on a raft. My body is demanding vigorous and regular workouts. There is one thing I refuse to resume, and that's dieting. Even if my health, age, or life circumstances conspire to pack on extra pounds (which, to date, they haven't), I have learned too much to consider anything as depriving and ineffective as a diet. For me, mindful eating is the only satisfying, effective way to go. Eating mindfully allows me to go to sleep satisfied and wake up hungry. If I do mindlessly eat past the point of comfortable fullness, I don't beat myself up, and I don't cut calories. Even if I'm bloated and irritable, I keep practicing self-compassion.

I have found good answers to the many questions that inspired my weight-loss journey. I don't pretend to have all the answers, but I do know this: food does not discriminate; it delivers pleasure and satisfaction to all takers. Satisfaction comes in a variety of portion sizes, as does pleasure. I can count on finding plenty of both when I take the time to notice what would hit the spot, and to shop, cook, set the table, fill my plate, sit, and savor the meal. I can also take sweet satisfaction in a quick bite without gobbling it up.

I have come to believe that where there's a will to stop and taste whatever you're eating, there's a sure way to arrive at your healthy, sustainable weight. Where there's genuine interest in cultivating mindful awareness and loving-kindness, there are real answers to the questions diet doctors can never answer for you. I'm quite certain that wherever you go on your weight-loss journey, you can count on finding satisfying answers in unexpected places—within yourself.

I don't love good-bye parties and other ceremonial obligations, but I do appreciate a heartfelt good-bye and a hypnotically poetic suggestion. Let me leave you with a little suggestion and a short good-bye for the road.

First, the suggestion:

Wherever you go,
my voice will go with you,
whispering words of loving-kindness.

Now, the good-bye:

> *May your journey be safe.*
> *May you travel in health and happiness.*
> *May you fare well.*

ACKNOWLEDGMENTS

Before writing this book, reading author acknowledgments made me more than a little envious. Most authors appeared to be rich in a priceless commodity: enthusiastic support. I had been in the writing business for more than three decades, and I had yet to realize the nose-on-face obvious truth: it takes a village or a *sangha,* as they say in meditation circles, to bring a book idea to bookstores. In writing *The Self-Compassion Diet,* I'd planned on studying the value of weight-loss support groups, but I hadn't expected to learn the importance of book-writing support. Like losing weight, I now know you gotta have sangha to write a book. Without it, you've got nothing but an interesting idea.

This book project also helped me acknowledge another under-acknowledged fact. Acknowledgements are not just for thanking those who have actively contributed to the writing effort, they're for recognizing helping hands from distant times and places, including typing fingers of kind strangers. I am brimming with appreciation for all supporters—my nearest and dearest who actively supported my best efforts up close and personal, as well as those who generously contributed from some distance.

The Self-Compassion Diet might have remained an interesting idea if it weren't for colleague-turned-mentor Chris Germer. Chris not only ignited my interest in self-compassion, he re-ignited my passion for bookwriting. If he'd never recited the *Bhagavad-Gita:* "It is better to do one's own duty, however defective it may be, than to follow the duty of another, however well one may perform it," or if he'd never sent his editor Kitty Moore my e-newsletter. Fact is, he did that and more. I've got Chris to thank for getting me started and keeping me up-to-date on all matters self-compassionate.

A book idea also needs a great agent to find a good publishing home. I'm grateful for the twenty agents who expressed interest and offered thoughtful criticism of the afore-titled *Slimming Lessons,* but I'm most grateful for dream agent Lindsay Edgecombe at Levine Greenberg Literary Agency. With intelligence, skill, and grace, this literary matchmaker fixed me up with the perfect publisher, Sounds True, and editor, Kelly Notaras. When Kelly stepped out, I'm thankful Haven Iverson stepped in. It's the rare editor who not only understands good writing and tonglen meditation, but wields a red pen, or should I say operates Track Changes, with loving-kindness.

Another rare breed is accomplished writers who are skillful teachers. I've had the good fortune of meeting two. Jon Lehman, my first editor, gave me a twofer chance of a young writer's lifetime: an entry-level position and a fitness column at my hometown newspaper. But the guy who taught me how to write clear, strong, attention-grabbing prose is the same guy who founded Harvard's Nieman Program on Narrative Journalism: Mark Kramer. Kramer deconstructed then reconstructed my personal essays—page by page, metaphor by metaphor, word by word. Thank you both.

The business of writing demands a different set of skills, and I was extremely fortunate to be tutored by the late, great Sarah Wernick, co-author of three bestselling fitness books. Her lessons on book-proposal writing, among other freelancing matters, were more than invaluable—they were quotable. My all-time favorite quote: "Don't squander your writing libido." She also introduced me to the ever-supportive, often witty writing organization that is the American Society of Journalists and Authors. Special shout-out to Kathy Seal,

Meg Lundstrom, and the wittiest of them all, Sophie Dembling. Heartfelt thanks also go to literary lawyer Sean Ploen.

The practice of psychotherapy calls for yet another set of skills and supporters. I've had the privilege of learning from an exceptional group of therapists in an extraordinary place—the department formerly known as the Behavioral Medicine Program at an institution previously called Cambridge Hospital. That the supervisors at this Harvard Medical School teaching affiliate are among the best and the brightest isn't what makes them exceptional. No, what makes guys like Peter McEntee and Larry Rosenberg extra-special is that they're humble and human. Despite their intelligence and talent, they're always ready to teach on demand and help in a pinch. I'm also thankful for the ongoing support of Peggy Kriss, Nicole Flory, and other members of the Advanced Behavioral Medicine Seminar. And the generous help of medical librarians Jenny Lee-Olsen and Patricia Redd.

Joy and Steve Gurgevich belong to a different team, but they're in the same league. Their loving and joyous support has been a gift. I also feel grateful to other generous supporters further afield, especially the researchers and writers who happily shared their work: Claire Adams, Gary Burlingame, LeeAnn Cardaciotto, Ken Goss, Jean Harvey-Berino, Paul Gilbert, Britta Hölzel, Jean Kristeller, Jim Sallis, Denise Wilfley, and Ruth Quillian Wolever.

Some of my best teachers are my clients. Their contributions on mindful, self-compassionate weight loss deserve public recognition, but their privacy needs protection. You know who you are. You're the ones who changed before my eyes and gave me the thumbs-up to share your success stories. But you've got no way of knowing your collective power. Your stories give life to this book and hope to despairing dieters everywhere. Thank you!

A good-sized thank you to my good friends and colleagues Rich Weintraub, Aline Zoldbrod, and my dear Alice Rosen. Tip of the lens cap to loyal friend and photographer Josh Touster. For their extraordinary care, a deep bow to Andrew Southcott, Miya Smith, and John Calabria.

More than a thank-you note, my family deserves a medal for making do with much less of me. My parents have more than earned medals of honor. My dad—for practicing what he preaches about diet and exercise. My mom—for loving words, and loving me more than words can say. Without her love and encouragement, my—I mean *our*—familial writing dreams would have never come true.

I can think of a few ways to thank my cat for standing or sitting by me, but how can I ever thank my devoted husband for staying calm, kind, and patient through the lengthy book-writing process? How can I possibly repay my multitalented guy for food shopping, cooking, and voluntarily providing other basic services, and freely offering professional computer support and insightful editorial advice. Given that he'd clearly rather be windsurfing than copyediting, I'm not sure I can. But I'm going to see what I can do.

NOTES

Chapter 1: The Kinder, Gentler Therapist

1. Kristin Neff's "Definition of Self-Compassion" is found at: self-compassion.org/what_is_self_compassion.html.
2. Kristin Neff, "Self-Compassion," in *Handbook of Individual Differences in Social Behavior,* ed. M. R. Leary and R. H. Hoyle (NY: Guilford Press, 2009), 561–73.
3. A. Lutz, J. Brefczynski-Lewis, T. Johnstone, and R. J. Davidson, "Regulation of the Neural Circuitry of Emotion by Compassion Meditation: Effects of Meditative Expertise," *PLoS ONE* 3, no. 3 (2008): 1–10.
4. Self-esteem information has been summarized from the following studies: M. R. Leary, E. B. Tate, C. E. Adams, A. B. Allen, and J. Hancock, "Self-Compassion and Reactions to Unpleasant Self-Relevant Events: The Implications of Treating Oneself Kindly," *Journal of Personality and Social Psychology* 92 (2007): 887–904; Neff, "Self-Compassion," 561–73; Kristin Neff, K. L. Kirkpatrick, S. S. Rude, and K. Dejitterat, "The Link between Self-Compassion and Psychological Well-Being," *Constructivism in the Human Sciences* 9, no. 2 (2004): 27–37; and Kristin Neff, "Self-Compassion: An Alternative Conceptualization of a Healthy Attitude toward Oneself," *Self and Identity* 2 (2003): 85–102.
5. Claire E. Adams and Mark R. Leary, "Promoting Self-Compassionate Attitudes toward Eating among Restrictive and

Guilty Eaters," *Journal of Social and Clinical Psychology* 26, no. 10 (2007): 1120–44.

6. Traci Mann, A. Janet Tomiyama, Erika Westling, Ann-Marie Lew, Barbra Samuels, and Jason Chatman, "Medicare's Search for Effective Obesity Treatments: Diets Are Not the Answer," *American Psychologist* 62, no. 3 (2007): 220–33.

7. Michelle Kirsch, "Be Kind to Yourself and Cure Your Eating Disorder," Timesonline.co.uk (April 18, 2007).

8. C. M. R. Magnus, "Does Self-Compassion Matter beyond Self-Esteem for Women's Self-Determined Motives to Exercise and Exercises Outcomes?" (master's thesis, University of Saskatchewan, Saskatoon, Canada, 2007).

9. Ellyn Satter, "What Is Normal Eating?" ellynsatter.com/ showArticle.jsp?id=268.

10. Kristin Neff, "Rate Your Self-Compassion Level," self-compassion.org/how_self-compassionate_are_you.html.

Chapter 2: Loving-Kindness Suggestions

1. Adapted from Kristin Neff, "Self-Compassion Scale for Researchers," webspace.utexas.edu/neffk/webpage/ Self_Compassion_Scale_for_researchers.doc; and Kristin Neff, "Development and Validation of a Scale to Measure Self-Compassion," *Self and Identity* 2 (2003): 223–50.

2. Narayan Liebenson Grady, "Guided Metta Meditation Dharma Talks," dharmaseed.org/teacher/131/?q=metta.

3. Christopher Germer, *The Mindful Path to Self-Compassion* (New York: Guilford, 2009).

4. Ken Goss, psychologist, Head of the Coventry Eating Disorders Services, in conversation with the author, 2008.

5. Adapted from the following sources: Paul Gilbert, "Building a Compassionate Guide," compassionatemind.co.uk/resources/

Building+a+compassionate+image$281$29.pdf; M. L. Rossman,
*Healing Yourself: A Step-by-Step Program for Better Health
through Imagery* (New York: Walker, 1987); Tara Brach, *Radical
Acceptance* (New York: Bantam, 2003).

6. Practice adapted from the following: Paul Gilbert,
   "Compassionate Letter Writing," compassionatemind.co.uk/
   resources/Compassionate+Letter+Writing$281$29.pdf; and
   Kristin Neff, "Exploring Self-Compassion through Writing,"
   self-compassion.org/exercises.doc.
7. Practice informed by Bart J. Walsh, "Hypnotic Alteration of
   Body Image in the Eating Disordered," *American Journal of
   Clinical Hypnosis* 50, no. 4 (2008): 301–10.
8. Practice informed by the following: Steven Gurgevich and Joy
   Gurgevich, *The Self-Hypnosis Diet* (Boulder, CO: Sounds True,
   2007); and Susie Orbach, *Fat Is a Feminist Issue I & II* (New
   York: Berkeley Books, 1978).
9. Practice informed by the following: Brach, *Radical Acceptance;*
   Pema Chödrön, *Awakening Loving-Kindness* (Boston: Shambhala
   Pocket Classics, 1996); and Pema Chödrön, "The Practice of
   Tonglen," shambhala.org/teachers/pema/tonglen1.php.

Chapter 3: The Enchanting Hypnotherapist

1. http://asch.net/genpubinfo.htm.
2. Informed by the following: Daniel P. Brown and Erika Fromm,
   Hypnotherapy and Hypnoanalysis (Hillsdale, NJ: Lawrence
   Erlbaum Associates, 1986); M. R. Nash and G. Benham, "The
   Truth and the Hype of Hypnosis," scientificamerican.com; and
   I. Kirsch and others, "Expectancy and Suggestibility: Are the
   Effects of Environmental Enhancement Due to Detection?" *The
   International Journal of Clinical and Experimental Hypnosis* 47
   (1999): 40–45.

3. G. Groth-Marnat and J. Schumaker, "Hypnotizability, Attitudes toward Eating, and Concern with Body Size in a Female College Population," *American Journal of Clinical Hypnosis* 32, no. 3 (1990): 194–200; and D. Thorne and others, "Are Fat Girls More Hypnotically Susceptible?" *Psychological Reports* 38, no. 1 (1976), 267–70.

4. Marianne Barabasz, "Efficacy of Hypnotherapy in the Treatment of Eating Disorders," *International Journal of Clinical and Experimental Hypnosis* 55, no. 3 (2007): 318–35.

5. I. Kirsch, G. Montgomery, and G. Sapirstein, "Hypnosis as an Adjunct to Cognitive Behavioral Psychotherapy: A Meta-Analysis," *Journal of Consulting and Clinical Psychology* 63 (1995): 214–20; and I. Kirsch, G. Montgomery, and G. Sapirstein, "Hypnotic Enhancement of Cognitive-Behavioral Weight Loss Treatments: Another Meta-Reanalysis," *Journal of Consulting and Clinical Psychology* 64: 517–519.

6. The National Weight Control Registry, nwcr.ws.

7. Sigmund Freud, *Hypnosis in The Standard Edition of the Complete Psychological Works of Sigmund Freud, Volume I (1886-1899): Pre-Psycho-Analytic Publications and Unpublished Drafts* (London: Hogarth Press, 1966), 103–14; and Rachel Bachner-Melman and P. Lichtenberg, "Freud's Relevance to Hypnosis: A Reevaluation," *American Journal of Clinical Hypnosis* 44, no. 1 (2001): 37–50.

8. Jacob H. Conn, "Historical Aspects of Scientific Hypnosis," *The International Journal of Clinical and Experimental Hypnosis* 5 (1957): 17–24; Samuel Glasner, "A Note on Allusions to Hypnosis in the Bible and Talmud," *The International Journal of Clinical and Experimental Hypnosis* 3 (1955): 34–39; and Arnold M. Ludwig, "An Historical Survey of the Early Roots of Mesmerism," *The International Journal of Clinical and Experimental Hypnosis* 12, no. 4 (1964): 205–17.

9. Steven J. Lynn and others, "Mindfulness, Acceptance, and Hypnosis: Cognitive and Clinical Perspectives," *The International Journal of Clinical and Experimental Hypnosis* 54, no. 2 (2006): 143–66.

10. Dave Foris, "The Effect of Meditation," *UW-L Journal of Undergraduate Research*, VIII (2005); and Amir Raz and others, "Suggestion Reduces the Stroop Effect," *Psychological Science* 17, no. 2 (2006): 91–95.

11. I. Kirsch, "Hypnotic Enhancement of Cognitive-Behavioral Weight Loss Treatments: Another Meta-Reanalysis," *Journal of Consulting and Clinical Psychology* 64 (1996): 517–19; and Ruth A. Baer, J. L. Kristeller, and R. Quillian-Wolever, "Mindfulness-Based Approaches to Eating Disorders," in *Mindfulness and Acceptance-Based Interventions: Conceptualization, Application, and Empirical Support*, ed. Ruth A. Baer (San Diego, CA: Elsevier, 2006), also available online at tcme.org/downloads/Baer%20Book-Ch4%20 eating%20Kristeller.pdf.

12. David N. Bolocofsky and others, "Effectiveness of Hypnosis as an Adjunct to Behavioral Weight Management," *Journal of Clinical Psychology* 41 (1985): 35–41.

Chapter 4: Winning Weight-loss Suggestions

1. Adapted from "Tellegen Absorption Scale," http://socrates. berkeley.edu/~kihlstrm/TAS.htm (John Kihlstrom's website).

2. D. Z. Cooper, C. G. Fairburn, and D. M. Hawker, *Cognitive-Behavioral Treatment of Obesity: A Clinician's Guide* (New York: Guilford, 2003), 129–45.

3. J. F. Hollis and others, "Weight Loss during the Intensive Intervention Phase of the Weight-Loss Maintenance Trial," *American Journal of Preventive Medicine* 35, no. 2 (2008): 118-26.

4. Michael Pollan, *In Defense of Food* (New York: Penguin Press, 2008).

5. Adapted from D. N. Bolocofsky and others, "Effectiveness of Hypnosis as an Adjunct to Behavioral Weight Management," *Journal of Clinical Psychology* 41 (1985): 35–41.

6. Adapted from H. Spiegel and D. Spiegel, *Trance and Treatment* (Arlington, VA: American Psychiatric Publishing, 2004).

7. Deirdre Barrett, psychologist, Harvard Medical School, in conversation with the author, 1999.

8. Informed by Brown and Fromm, *Hypnosis and Behavioral Medicine.*

Chapter 5: The Curious Meditator

1. "Integrating Mindfulness-Based Interventions into Medicine, Health Care, and Society," UMass Medical School's Center for Mindfulness conference (2005); and Ruth Wolever and J. Best, "Mindfulness-Based Approaches," in *Clinical Handbook of Mindfulness,* ed. F. Didonna (New York: Springer, 2009), 259–88.

2. Jean Kristeller, "Mindful Weight Loss: Inner Wisdom and Outer Wisdom," *Food for Thought: A Quarterly Newsletter from the Center for Mindful Eating* (Winter 2010): 1–3, tcme.org.

3. Ruth Wolever and others, "Determining the Effects of Mindfulness Based Weight Loss Maintenance (MBWLM) on a Key Inflammatory Marker, Interleukin-6" and "Mindfulness in the Maintenance of Weight Loss: A Randomized Controlled Trial of EMPOWER program" (abstracts, 2010).

4. Kenneth P. Wright, "Too Little Sleep: A Risk Factor for Obesity?" *Obesity Management* 2, no. 4 (2006): 140–45; and Jean Kristeller, innovator of Mindfulness-Based Eating Awareness Training, in conversation with the author, 2005.

5. Reverend H. Sure, "On Fasting from a Buddhist's Perspective," urbandharma.org/udharma9/fasting.html.

6. Kristeller, conversation.

7. Orbach, *Fat Is a Feminist Issue.*

8. Renee Lertzman, "An Interview with Geneen Roth on Mindful-Eating," *The Sun* 313 (2002), thesunmagazine.org/issues/313.

9. Mireille Guiliano, *French Women Don't Get Fat* (New York: Knopf, 2005).

10. Richard W. Schwarz, *John Harvey Kellogg: Pioneering Health Reformer* (Hagerstown, MD: Review and Herald, 2006); and Wikipedia: http://en.wikipedia.org/wiki/John_Harvey_Kellogg.

11. "Mindfulness and Psychotherapy," conference at Harvard Medical School (2009).

12. Kirk W. Brown, R. M. Ryan, and J. D. Creswell, "Mindfulness: Theoretical Foundations and Evidence for Its Salutary Effects," *Psychological Inquiry* 18, no. 4 (2007): 211–37.

13. Baer and others, "Mindfulness-Based Approaches," 1–32 (also at: tcme.org/downloads/Baer%20Book-Ch4%20eating%20 Kristeller.pdf); and Ruth Wolever and J. Best, "Mindfulness-Based Approaches to Eating Disorders," in *Clinical Handbook of Mindfulness,* ed. F. Didonna (New York: Springer, 2009), 259–88.

14. E. M. Forman and others, "An Open Trial of an Acceptance-Based Behavioral Intervention for Weight Loss," *Cognitive and Behavioral Practice* 16, no. 2 (2009): 223–35.

15. Koutatsu Maruyama and others, "The Joint Impact on Being Overweight of Self Reported Behaviours of Eating Quickly and Eating Until Full: Cross Sectional Survey," *British Medical Journal Online* (October 21, 2008), bmj.com/cgi/content/full/337/oct21_2/a2002.

16. Nirbhay N. Singh and others, "A Mindfulness-Based Health Wellness Program for Managing Morbid Obesity," *Clinical Case Studies* 7, no. 4 (2008): 327–39.

17. Informed by the following sources: Richard J. Davidson,

J. Kabat-Zinn, and others, "Alterations in Brain and Immune Function Produced by Mindfulness Meditation," *Psychosomatic Medicine* 65, no. 4 (2003): 564–70; Sara W. Lazar, "Mindfulness Research," in *Mindfulness and Psychotherapy*, ed. Christopher Germer, R. D. Siegel, and P. R. Fulton (New York: Guilford, 2005), 220–38; Christopher Germer, *The Mindful Path to Self-Compassion* (New York: Guilford, 2009).

18. "Integrating Mindfulness-Based Interventions," conference, 2005.

19. Britta Hölzel and U. Ott, "Relationships between Meditation Depth, Absorption, Meditation Practice, and Mindfulness: A Latent Variable Approach," *Journal of Transpersonal Psychology* 38, no. 2 (2006): 179–99.

20. David Engstrom, "Eating Mindfully and Cultivating Satisfaction: Modifying Eating Patterns in a Bariatric Surgery Patient" in *Bariatric Nursing and Surgical Patient Care* 2, no. 4 (2007): 245–50; and Karen Ballen, "Mindful Eating: An Interview with Dr. David Engstrom," in *Bariatric Nursing and Surgical Patient Care* 2, no. 4 (2007): 237–43.

21. L. D. Levy, J. P. Fleming, and D. Klar, "Treatment of Refractory Obesity in Severely Obese Adults Following Management of Newly Diagnosed ADHD," *International Journal of Obesity* 33 (2009): 326–34.

22. Yi-Yuan Tang and others, "Short-Term Meditation Training Improves Attention and Self-Regulation," *PNAS: Proceedings of the National Academy of Sciences of the United States of America* 104, no. 43 (2007): 17152–56.

23. *People Magazine* 70, no. 7 (Aug. 18, 2008), people.com/people/archive/article/0,,20221739,00.html.

24. Thich Nhat Hanh, "Mindful Eating," *Chet Day's Health & Beyond,* http://chetday.com/mindfuleating.htm.

Chapter 6: Mindful Eating Suggestions

1. Adapted from the following sources: Celia Framson and others, "Development and Validation of the Mindful Eating Questionnaire," *Journal of the American Dietetic Association* 109, no. 8 (2009): 1439–44; and L. Cardaciotto, "The Assessment of Present-Moment Awareness and Acceptance: The Philadelphia Mindfulness Scale," *Assessment* 15, no. 2 (2008): 204–23.

2. Brian Wansink, *Mindless Eating* (New York: Bantam Books, 2006).

Chapter 7: The Successful Weight-Loss Buddy

1. Caroline Knapp, *Pack of Two* (New York: Delta, 1998).

2. Informed by the following: Irwin G. Sarason and others, "Assessing Social Support: The Social Support Questionnaire," *Journal of Personality and Social Psychology* 44, no. 1 (1983): 127–39; and James F. Sallis and others, "The Development of Scales to Measure Social Support for Diet and Exercise Behaviors," *Preventive Medicine* 16, no. 6 (1987): 825–36.

3. Informed by several sources including: Gary M. Burlingame and D. T. McClendon, "Group Therapy," in *Twenty-First-Century Psychotherapies*, ed. J. L. Lebow (Hoboken, NJ: John Wiley & Sons, 2008), 347–88; Gary Burlingame and S. Baldwin, "History of Group Psychotherapy," in *History of Psychotherapy*, ed. J. Norcross, G. VandenBos, and D. Freedheim, 2nd ed. (Washington DC: American Psychological Association, 2010); and Dianne Hales and Robert E. Hales, *Caring for the Mind* (New York: Bantam, 1995).

4. Irvin Yalom and Molyn Leszcz, *The Theory and Practice of Group Psychotherapy* (New York: Basic Books, 2005).

5. G. Terence Wilson and K. D. Brownell, "Behavioral Treatment for Obesity," in *Eating Disorders and Obesity*, ed. Christopher G. Fairburn and Kelly D. Brownell, 2nd ed. (New York: Guilford, 2002), 524–28.

6. Adam G. Tsai and T. A. Wadden, "Systematic Review: An Evaluation of the Major Commercial Weight Loss Programs in the U.S.," *Annals of Internal Medicine* 142 (2005): 56–66.

7. National Weight Control Registry, nwcr.ws/Research/default.htm.

8. Michael G. Perri, "Improving Maintenance in Behavioral Treatment" in "Eating Disorders and Obesity" ed. Christopher G. Fairburn and Kelly D. Brownell, 2nd ed. (New York: Guilford, 2002), 593–598; Janet D. Latner and others, "The Perceived Effectiveness of Continuing Care and Group Support in the Long-Term Self-Help Treatment of Obesity," *Obesity* 14, no. 3 (2006): 464–71; and Robert W. Jeffery and others, "Long-Term Maintenance of Weight Loss: Current Status," *Health Psychology* 19, no. 1 (2000): 5–16.

9. Amy Gorin, S. Phelan, D. Tate, N. Sherwood, R. Jeffery, and R. Wing, "Involving Support Partners in Obesity Treatment," *Journal of Consulting and Clinical Psychology* 73, no. 2 (2005): 341–43.

10. Clive Thompson, "Are Your Friends Making You Fat?" *New York Times Magazine*, nytimes.com/2009/09/13/magazine/13contagion-t.html?pagewanted=all.

11. Tsai and Wadden, "Commercial Weight Loss Programs," 56–66.

12. Wilson and Brownell, "Behavioral Treatment for Obesity," 524–28; and Jeffery and others, "Long-Term Maintenance of Weight Loss," 5–16.

13. Carol B. Peterson and others, "The Efficacy of Self-Help Group Treatment and Therapist-Led Group Treatment for Binge Eating Disorder," *American Journal of Psychiatry* 166, no. 12 (2009): 1347–54.

14. D. A. Renjilian and others, "Individual versus Group Therapy for Obesity: Effects of Matching Participants to Their Treatment Preferences," *Journal of Consulting and Clinical Psychology* 69, no. 4 (2001): 717–21.

15. David R. Black, L. J. Gleser, and K. J. Kooyers, "A Meta-Analytic Evaluation of Couples Weight-Loss Programs," *Health Psychology* 9, no. 3 (1990): 330–47.

16. R. R. Wing and R. W. Jeffery, "Benefits of Recruiting Participants with Friends and Increasing Social Support for Weight Loss and Maintenance," *Journal of Consulting and Clinical Psychology* 67, no. 1 (1999): 132–38.

17. Kelly D. Brownell and others, "Weight Loss Competitions at the Work Site: Impact on Weight, Morale and Cost-Effectiveness," *American Journal Public Health* 74 (1984): 1283–85.

18. Louisa Kasdon, "Party of 12: A Real Women's Weight-Loss Group," *More* (March 2007), more.com/2030/3140-party-of-12-a-real.

19. Robert F. Kushner, D. J. Blatner, D. E. Jewell, and K. Rudloff, "The PPET Study: People and Pets Exercising Together," *Obesity* 14, no. 10 (2006): 1762–70.

20. Informed by the following sources: Kevin R. Fontaine and D. B. Allison, "Obesity and the Internet," in *Eating Disorder and Obesity,* ed. C. G. Fairburn and K. D. Brownell, 2nd ed. (New York: Guilford, 2002), 609–12; N. L. Atkinson and R. S. Gold, "The Promise and Challenge of eHealth Interventions," *American Journal of Health Behavior* 26 (2002), 494–503; and Nicci Micco and others, "Minimal In-Person Support as an Adjunct to Internet Obesity Treatment," *Annals of Behavioral Medicine* 33, no. 1 (2007): 49–56.

21. Beth C. Gold, S. Burke, S. Pintauro, P. Buzzell, and J. Harvey-Berino, "Weight Loss on the Web: A Pilot Study Comparing a Structured Behavioral Intervention to a Commercial Program," *Obesity* 15, no. 1 (2007): 155–64.

22. Pamela M. Grayson, "Put Your Money Where Your Fat Is," *New York Times,* nytimes.com/2009/02/05/health/nutrition/05fitness.html.

Chapter 8: Seeking Support

1. James Prochaska, J. Norcross, and C. DiClemente, *Changing for Good* (New York: Avon Books, 1994).
2. Adapted from James F. Sallis and others, "The Development of Scales to Measure Social Support for Diet and Exercise," *Preventive Medicine* 16, no. 6 (1987): 825–36.
3. Deirdre Barrett, *Waistland: The (R)Evolutionary Science Behind Our Weight and Fitness Crisis* (New York: Norton, 2007).

Chapter 9: Filling Your Toolbox

1. Leonard Pearson, *The Psychologist's Eat-Anything Diet* (New York: P. H. Wyden, 1973).

FURTHER READING
AND RESOURCES

We shall not cease from exploration
And the end of all our exploring
Will be to arrive where we started
And know the place for the first time.

T. S. ELIOT

When the shiny, new tool-set that is *The Self-Compassion Diet* gets comfortably worn with use, you may want to add additional tools to the set. If and when you find yourself in the market for a new something-or-other, you could probably use a few good recommendations or a list of further reading and resources like this one. The dizzying number of available weight-loss products and services can make your head spin, but this section aims to have the opposite effect—to inspire a calm focus, to help you steadily continue your education and exploration of the four weight-loss routes: compassion, mindfulness, hypnosis, and social support.

Before I share a few of my favorite books, CDs, and websites, I'd like to share a few words on why I listed this and not that, here and not there. Because mindfulness and self-compassion are kind of inseparable, creating a separate category for each was no easy task. But to make it easier for you to take the next step on your journey, I was determined to divide and conquer. Many resources belong in both categories, but I was also set on saving a little space and a few trees. So I put anything with a loving-kindness focus in the Self-Compassion category, and all things food-focused under Mindful Eating. I also recommended no more than ten books per category for the first three categories, and not a one for the last. If you're in the market for social support, what you really need is people, not books.

Therefore, under Social Support, the only resources you'll find are human resources, online and in-person options for meeting like-minded waist watchers. As you know, I'm not a big fan of diets, but if you're in a dieting state of mind, that's where you are. To help you do what every waist watcher needs to do—weigh your best options—I've listed several diet organizations. Finally, if you're in need of professional help, I've offered route-by-route suggestions for finding the help you need in the form of NSQs (No Stupid Questions).

That's all you really need to know right now. Ready to continue your exploration?

SELF-COMPASSION
Books

Allione, Tsultrim. *Feeding Your Demons: Ancient Wisdom for Resolving Inner Conflict.* New York: Little Brown, 2008.

Brach, Tara. *Radical Acceptance: Embracing Your Life with the Heart of a Buddha.* New York: Bantam, 2003.

Chödrön, Pema. *Awakening Loving-Kindness.* Boston: Shambhala, 1991.

———. *Start Where You Are: A Guide to Compassionate Living.* Boston: Shambhala, 2001.

Germer, Christopher K. *The Mindful Path to Self-Compassion: Freeing Yourself from Destructive Thoughts and Emotions.* New York: Guilford, 2009.

Hanh, Thich Nhat. *Teachings on Love.* Berkeley: Parallax Press, 1997.

Salzberg, Sharon. *Lovingkindness: The Revolutionary Art of Happiness.* Boston: Shambhala, 2002.

————. *The Force of Kindness: Change Your Life with Love and Compassion.* Boulder, CO: Sounds True, 2005.

————. *The Kindness Handbook: A Practical Companion.* Boulder, CO: Sounds True, 2008.

Audio CDs

Fain, Jean. *Compassionate Weight Loss: A Jean Fain Mindfulness CD.* Concord, MA: Jean Fain, 2009.

Hanh, Thich Nhat. *The Art of Mindful Living: How to Bring Love, Compassion, and Inner Peace into Your Daily Life.* Boulder, CO: Sounds True, 2000.

Salzberg, Sharon. *Guided Meditations for Love and Wisdom.* Boulder, CO: Sounds True, 2009.

————. *Lovingkindness Meditation: Learning to Love through Insight Meditation.* Boulder, CO: Sounds True, 2004.

Online Resources

Tara Brach's website: tarabrach.com

Pema Chödrön's online offerings: shambhala.org/teachers/pema/tonglen1.php, pemachodrontapes.org

The Compassionate Mind Foundation: compassionatemind.co.uk

The Dalai Lama's website: dalailama.com

Dharma Seed's recorded meditation teachings and practices: dharmaseed.org

Jean Fain's YouTube Channel: *Compassionate Weight Loss.* youtube.com/watch?v=_a05ACO8QPE

Kristin Neff's self-compassion website: self-compassion.org

Mind & Life Institute: mindandlife.org

Mindful Self-Compassion recorded meditations: mindfulselfcompassion.org/meditations_downloads.php

Sharon Salzberg's website: sharonsalzberg.com

The Center for Compassion and Altruism Research and Education: http://ccare.stanford.edu/

Thich Nhat Hanh's online offerings: iamhome.org, plumvillage.org

MINDFUL EATING
Books

Albers, Susan. *Eat, Drink, and Be Mindful: How to End Your Struggle with Mindless Eating and Start Savoring Food with Intention and Joy.* Oakland, CA: New Harbinger, 2009.

Antonello, Jean. *Breaking Out of Food Jail: How to Free Yourself from Diets and Problem Eating, Once and for All.* New York: Fireside, 1996.

Craighead, Linda. *The Appetite Awareness Workbook: How to Listen to Your Body & Overcome Bingeing, Overeating & Obsessions with Food.* Oakland, CA: New Harbinger, 2006.

David, Mark. *The Slow Down Diet: Eating for Pleasure, Energy, & Weight Loss.* Rochester, VT: Healing Arts Press, 2005.

Gerrard, Don. *One Bowl: A Guide to Eating for Body and Spirit.* New York: Marlowe & Company, 1974.

Orbach, Susie. *Fat is a Feminist Issue: The Anti-Diet Guide to Permanent Weight Loss.* Edison, NJ: BBS Publishing Corporation, 2007.

Pollan, Michael. *In Defense of Food: An Eater's Manifesto.* New York: Penguin, 2008.

Roth, Geneen. *Women, Food, and God: An Unexpected Path to Almost Anything.* New York: Scribner, 2010.

Satter, Ellyn. *How to Get Your Kid to Eat . . . But Not Too Much.* Boulder, CO: Bull Publishing Company, 1987.

Tribole, Evelyn, and Elyse Resch. *Intuitive Eating: A Revolutionary Program that Works.* New York: St. Martin's Press, 1995.

Audio CDs

Fain, Jean. *Eating Awareness Training: A Jean Fain Mindfulness CD.* Concord, MA: Jean Fain, 2006.

———. *Mindful Eating: A Jean Fain Mindfulness CD.* Concord, MA: Jean Fain, 2005.

———. *The Self-Compassion Diet: Guided Practices to Lose Weight with Loving-Kindness.* Boulder, CO: Sounds True, 2011.

Kabat-Zinn, Jon. *Guided Mindfulness Meditation: Series 1, 2, and 3.* Lexington, MA: Jon Kabat-Zinn, 2002, 2003, and 2005.

Rosen, Alice. *The Feeding Ourselves Method: A Guide to Achieving a Healthy Relationship with Food.* Concord, MA: Alice Rosen, 2004.

Roth, Geneen. *Bite by Bite: Seven Guidelines to Break Free from Emotional Eating.* Boulder, CO: Sounds True, 2006.

———. *Feeding The Hungry Heart: An Audio Workshop on Healing Your Relationship with Food.* Boulder, CO: Sounds True, 2005.

———. *When Food Is Food and Love Is Love.* Boulder, CO: Sounds True, 2005.

Tribole, Evelyn, and Elyse Resch. *Intuitive Eating.* Boulder, CO: Sounds True, 2009.

NO STUPID QUESTIONS

Q I'd love to find a compassionate psychotherapist. Any suggestions for how to find one?

A Although there are good therapy referral services (you'll find a few under Social Supports), there's no database of compassionate therapists. Even if there were, it could only tell you who's studied or meditated on compassion. In theory, all therapists are trained to listen with a compassionate ear. In practice, the ability to listen varies greatly between therapists and within the same therapist over time. The best way to find a compassionate therapist is to consult one or more. Sit and talk. See how it feels. If you come away feeling listened to, cared for, respected, you may have found your compassionate therapist. If you're left with a less favorable impression, try another couch. See how it feels.

Weil, Andrew. *Healthy Eating: Dr. Andrew Weil on Eating for Optimum Health and Pleasure.* Boulder, CO: Sounds True, 2003.

Online Resources

Susan Albers' Eat, Drink, and Be Mindful: eatingmindfully.com

The Center for Mindful Eating: tcme.org

The Conscious Cafe: theconsciouscafe.org

eMindful: emindful.com

Michael Pollan's website: michaelpollan.com

The Mindfulness Solution's recorded meditations: mindfulness-solution.com/DownloadMeditations.html

Geneen Roth's website: geneenroth.com

Ellyn Satter's website: ellynsatter.com

Slow Food International: slowfood.com

HYPNOSIS

Books

Alman, Brian. *Keep It Off: Use the Power of Self-Hypnosis to Lose Weight Now.* New York: Dutton, 2004.

Alman, Brian, and Peter Lambrou. *Self-Hypnosis: The Complete Manual for Health and Self-Change.* 2nd ed. New York: Brunner-Routledge, 1992.

Barrett, Deirdre. *Waistland: The (R)Evolutionary Science Behind Our Weight and Fitness Crisis.* New York: Norton, 2007.

Fisher, Stanley. *Discovering the Power of Self-Hypnosis: The Simple, Natural Mind-Body Approach to Change and Healing.* New York: Newmarket Press, 1991.

Gurgevich, Steven, and Joy Gurgevich. *The Self-Hypnosis Diet: Use the Power of Your Mind to Reach Your Perfect Weight.* Boulder, CO: Sounds True, 2007.

Hammond, D. Corydon. *Manual for Self-Hypnosis*. Des Plaines, IL: American Society of Clinical Hypnosis, 1992.

Rosen, Sidney. *My Voice Will Go with You: The Teaching Tales of Milton H. Erickson*. New York: Norton, 1991.

Temes, Roberta. *The Complete Idiot's Guide to Hypnosis*. 2nd ed. New York: Alpha Books, 2004.

Audio CDs

Alman, Brian. *Keep It Off: Use the Power of Self-Hypnosis to Lose Weight Now.* selfhypnosis.com: Brian Alman, 2004.

Fain, Jean. *Eat to Live & Lose Weight: A Jean Fain Hypnosis CD.* Concord, MA: Jean Fain, 2005.

———. *Mindful Eating Mini Trances: A Jean Fain Hypnosis CD.* Concord, MA: Jean Fain, 2007.

Gurgevich, Steven. *The Self-Hypnosis Diet: Use the Power of Your Mind to Make Any Diet Work for You.* Boulder, CO: Sounds True, 2006.

NO STUPID QUESTIONS

Q How do I find a mindful-eating therapist?

A Until there's a therapy referral service that specializes in mindful eating, you'll need to conduct a private investigation. See if you can turn up a referral from your physician, therapist, anyone in the know. You might also investigate a group practice or alliance of therapists that specializes in mindfulness-based psychotherapy, like Boston's renowned Institute for Meditation and Psychotherapy (meditationandpsychotherapy. org). Even if you don't have a diagnosable eating disorder, you may be able to track down a qualified therapist through an eating-disorder referral service. Many eating-disorder experts also treat yo-yo dieting and other everyday eating issues. Ideally, you'll find a therapist experienced in your particular eating issue and trained in one of the mindfulness-based therapies described in chapter 5. Realistically, if you live far from an epicenter of mindfulness training and research, you may have to widen your search to include any and all psychotherapists who practice mindfulness. Or check out your virtual options for telephone and online therapy.

Q How do I find a trustworthy hypnotherapist for weight loss?

A Visit the website of the Societies of Hypnosis (societiesofhypnosis.com). There you'll find a referral database of hypnosis professionals in psychotherapy, medicine, and dentistry around the world. Look for a mental health professional (psychiatrist, psychologist, social worker) who's trained in hypnotherapy and specializes in eating issues. (It's even better if the therapist is also schooled in self-compassion.)

Gurgevich, Steven, and Joy Gurgevich. *Lose Weight with Hypnosis: Nourishing Mind and Body for Healthy Weight.* Tuscon, AZ: Tranceformation Works, 2002.

Temes, Roberta. *Enjoying Weight Loss.* hypnosisnetwork.com: The Hypnosis Network, 2005.

Online Resources

American Society of Clinical Hypnosis: asch.net

Jean Fain's YouTube Channel: *Mindful Eating Trance.* youtube.com/watch?v=ROltyC6-Glw

―――. *Mindless Eating Trance.* youtube.com/user/jeanfain#p/a/f/1/yOaMzFsLk9M

―――. *Why a Twinkie?* youtube.com/user/jeanfain#p/a/f/0/egMjE1_YGII

Steven Gurgevich and Joy Gurgevich's website: tranceformation.com/mainh.html

Society for Clinical & Experimental Hypnosis: netforum.avectra.com/eWeb/StartPage.aspx?Site=SCEH

New England Society of Clinical Hypnosis: nesch.org

Societies of Hypnosis: societiesofhypnosis.com

Telegen Absorption Scale: socrates.berkeley.edu/~kihlstrm/TAS.htm

SOCIAL SUPPORT

Online Resources: Nonprofessional

Diet Organizations

eDiets: ediets.com

Jenny Craig Weight Loss Program: jennycraig.com

LA Weight Loss: la-weightloss.com

Overeaters Anonymous: oa.org

TOPS (Take Off Pounds Sensibly):
  tops.org

Weight Watchers: WeightWatchers.com

Dieting and Diet-Betting Websites

Bitch Yourself Thin:
  bitchyourselfthin.com

Fat Bet: fatbet.net

Hungry Girl: hungry-girl.com

Make Money Losing Weight:
  makemoneylosingweight.com

StickK: stickK.com

Healthy Eating / Cooking / Living Blogs

Beautiful You By Julie:
  beautifulyoubyjulie.com

Eat without Guilt:
  eatwithoutguilt.com

101 Cookbooks: 101cookbooks.com

Skinny Scoopers: skinnyscoopers.com

You'd Be So Pretty If . . . :
  youdbesoprettyif.com

Online Resources: Professional Obesity Organizations

American Dietetic Association: eatright.org

CDC's Healthy Weight:
  cdc.gov/healthyweight

NO STUPID QUESTIONS

Q I know I need support, but I've never found diet groups all that supportive. Where can I find a group I can call my own?

A Before you ask around for recommendations, I encourage you to look within for answers. If you've yet to try the practices in chapter 8, why not start there? The writing exercises and visualizations will help you remember whose support proved helpful before, and what kind of help would be most useful now. The simplest thing you can do, of course, is to pay attention. Notice which weight-loss supports pique your interest. Listen to what successful waist watchers are saying about their winning weight-loss team. If group therapy sounds appealing, consider asking your health-care provider for a referral, or consulting a therapy referral service. Keep asking around and looking within. If you don't find what you're looking for, you just might have to get together with like-minded waist watchers and create your own group.

National Weight Control Registry: nwcr.ws

The Obesity Society: obesity.org

Shape Up America!: shapeup.org

Psychotherapy Referral Services

Eating Disorder Referral and Information Center: edreferral.com

GoodTherapy.org: goodtherapy.org

HelpPro Therapist Finder: helppro.com

Multi-service Eating Disorders Association: medainc.org

National Eating Disorders Association: nationaleatingdisorders.org

Psychology Today Therapy Directory:
    therapists.psychologytoday.com/rms/

Something Fishy Website on Eating Disorders: something-fishy.org

Academic Resources

The Center for Mindfulness in Medicine, Health Care, and Society:
    umassmed.edu/cfm/home/index.aspx

The Cooper Institute: standupandeat.org

Duke Integrative Medicine: dukeintegrativemedicine.org

Harvard School of Public Health: thenutritionsource.org, and
    hsph.harvard.edu/prc

Dr. James Sallis's Eating and Exercise Surveys: drjamessallis.sdsu.
    edu/Documents/socialsupport-eatinghabits.pdf, and
    drjamessallis.sdsu.edu/Documents/socialsupport-exercise.pdf

VTrim Online Weight-Management Program: uvm.edu/vtrim

Other Websites

BeWell Healthy Conversations Online: bewell.com

Have Your Cake and Eat It Too: rivkasimmons.com

Mollie Katzen's website: molliekatzen.com
Karen Koenig's online offerings: eatingnormal.com,
   eatingdisordersblogs.com/healthy/

ABOUT THE AUTHOR

Whether she's teaching at Harvard Medical School, seeing clients in her private practice, or writing for magazines, Jean Fain, LICSW, is dedicated to helping people keep physically, emotionally and mentally fit. As a teaching associate in psychiatry at Cambridge Health Alliance, a teaching affiliate of Harvard Medical School, she teaches hypnosis and mind-body medicine to physicians, psychologists, and social workers. Entering the third decade of her career as a psychotherapist and reflecting on the variety of settings she's worked in—state prisons, community mental health centers, rape crisis centers, public hospitals—she considers it a great privilege and pleasure to see clients solely in her Concord, Massachusetts, private practice.

Jean's writing career predates her clinical practice. A veteran journalist, you may have seen her articles in *O: The Oprah Magazine, Condé Nast Traveler, Shape,* the *Boston Globe,* or the *Los Angeles Times* syndicate. Writing about physical and mental health for magazines and newspapers allows her to reach people beyond the scope of her small therapy practice.

Jean lives with her husband and cat in the heart of Thoreau country surrounded by farms, woods, and rivers. She lives a stone's throw from Walden Pond State Reservation, but you won't find her at that literary landmark during tourist season. No, you're more likely to find her at the neighborhood farm stand, hiking off the beaten path, or swimming across one of the lesser-known ponds. Or you might find her tending to the backyard garden, or in the kitchen cooking up something delicious and nutritious. Wherever she happens to be, you can always learn more about Jean on her website at jeanfain.com.

ABOUT SOUNDS TRUE

Sounds True is a multimedia publisher whose mission is to inspire and support personal transformation and spiritual awakening. Founded in 1985 and located in Boulder, Colorado, we work with many of the leading spiritual teachers, thinkers, healers, and visionary artists of our time. We strive with every title to preserve the essential "living wisdom" of the author or artist. It is our goal to create products that not only provide information to a reader or listener, but that also embody the quality of a wisdom transmission.

For those seeking genuine transformation, Sounds True is your trusted partner. At SoundsTrue.com you will find a wealth of free resources to support your journey, including exclusive weekly audio interviews, free downloads, interactive learning tools, and other special savings on all our titles.

To learn more, please visit SoundsTrue.com/bonus/free_gifts or call us toll free at 800.333.9185.

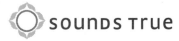

SOUNDS TRUE

PO Box 8010
Boulder CO 80306